Essential Lists of Differential Diagnoses for MRCP

with diagnostic hints

FAZAL-I-AKBAR DANISH

CT2 in Medicine
Princess of Wales Hospital, Bridgend

Radcliffe Publishing
Oxford • New York

To Iman.

Radcliffe Publishing Ltd
18 Marcham Road
Abingdon
Oxon OX14 1AA
United Kingdom

www.radcliffe-oxford.com

Electronic catalogue and worldwide online ordering facility.

British Library Cataloguing in Publication Data

A catalogue record for this book is available from the British Library.

ISBN-13: 978 184619 421 4

The paper used for the text pages of this book is FSC certified. FSC (The Forest Stewardship Council) is an international network to promote responsible management of the world's forests.

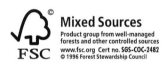

Mixed Sources
Product group from well-managed forests and other controlled sources
www.fsc.org Cert no. SGS-COC-2482
© 1996 Forest Stewardship Council

Typeset by Pindar NZ, Auckland, New Zealand
Printed and bound by TJI Digital, Padstow, Cornwall, UK

Contents

Preface

This book is distinct from other books on the same subject in the sense that I have tried to refrain from burdening my readers with long and exhausting lists of (rare) causes. Instead, I have tried to restrict most of the lists to a maximum of five items that constitute the most common causes in terms of disease prevalence. This strategy is intended to help candidates not only pass the postgraduate exams but also to become competent clinicians (patient has metabolic acidosis, think of uraemia or DKA instead of paraldehyde toxicity).

Additionally, I have included what I call 'Diagnostic hints'. These refer to clinical or lab clues that if present in a clinical scenario point towards a specific diagnosis (e.g. mouth and genital ulcers, think of Behçet's syndrome, etc.).

I have also included a chapter on ECG – something that I believe is unique. It contains lists of causes of ECG changes (e.g. causes of T wave inversion, hyperacute T waves, prolonged PR interval, etc.) and, conversely, key ECG features of common diagnoses (e.g. atrial fibrillation, MI, AV block, etc.).

The book is primarily intended for MRCP (UK) (both Part I and Part II) and FCPS (Pakistan) (Part II) candidates, although it may also be helpful for undergraduate students preparing for their finals.

Fazal-I-Akbar Danish
January 2010

Contributors

Salman S Koul MBBS FCPS-I (Pak) MCPS (Pak)
Registrar
Department of Medicine
Pakistan Institute of Medical Sciences (PIMS)
Islamabad, Pakistan

Fazal R Subhani MBBS FCPS-I (Pak)
Registrar
Department of Paediatrics
Holy Family Hospital
Rawalpindi, Pakistan

Ahmed E Rabbani
Final Year Medical Student
Foundation University Medical College (FUMC)
Rawalpindi, Pakistan

Saeeda Yasmin MBBS FCPS (Pak) MRCS (UK)
Consultant Surgeon
Shifa Hospital
Islamabad, Pakistan

About the author

Dr Fazal graduated from Army Medical College, Rawalpindi, Pakistan in 1999. After working in his home country for a few years in various capacities, he shifted to the UK in 2005 and has worked as Clinical Research Fellow in the Universities of Southampton and Bristol, and as a Medical SHO in various NHS trusts. Although a junior doctor, Dr Fazal has contributed appreciably in medical literature. He is the first and corresponding author of eight research papers published in different peer-reviewed journals. He has contributed a 28-web-page section namely 'Phenotyping' in an online encyclopaedia entitled 'Online Encyclopedia for Genetic Epidemiology Studies', www.oege.org. This section links and describes standardised research protocols and related information for clinical phenotyping of common diseases and risk traits. It is primarily of relevance to researchers and PhD students. Dr Fazal has three medical books to his credit – the book in your hand, *Hospital Dermatology* (a 226-page book for final year medical students and postgraduate trainees) and *Pharmacology in 7 Days for Medical Students* (a 166-page book for third year medical students). He is currently working as a CT2 in Medicine at the Princess of Wales Hospital in Bridgend.

1 General physical examination

Thin, wasted, cachectic:
1 Low calorie intake (d/t anorexia nervosa; alcoholism; drug abuse; prolonged systemic illness, e.g. COPD).
2 Tuberculosis.
3 Malignancy.
4 Thyrotoxicosis.
5 AIDS.

Fingernail abnormalities:
1 Clubbing. Acute/chronic paronychia.
2 Nail fold infarcts (d/t vasculitis).
3 Lines (Beau's; longitudinal; Muehrcke's; Mee's; Terry's).
4 Splinter haemorrhages.
5 Yellow nails.
6 Nail pitting.
7 Koilonychia.
8 Onycholysis.
9 Onychomadesis (shedding of nail).

Clubbing:
1 Respiratory disease (malignancy; infection [lung abscess, empyema]; bronchiectasis; fibrosing alveolitis).
2 Cardiac disease (congenital cyanotic heart disease [Fallot's tetralogy, transposition of the great arteries]; acyanotic heart disease, i.e. PDA with 'reversal of shunt' [clubbing only in the toes]; infective endocarditis).
3 Subclavian artery aneurysm (clubbing is unilateral).
4 GIT disease (cirrhosis; PBC; IBD; malabsorption – coeliac disease, Whipple's disease).

Cyanosis (non-oxygenated Hb >5 g/dL):
1 Peripheral cyanosis:[1]
   a Shock (hypovolaemic; cardiogenic; septic d/t gram-negative organisms usually).
   b Cold weather (Raynaud's phenomenon).
   c Arterial/venous occlusion (d/t atheroma or small-vessel disease in diabetes).

---

1 Fingers, hands, nose, cheeks and ears would be cold and bluish.

2 Central cyanosis:[2]
  a Respiratory failure.
  b Congenital heart disease (Fallot's tetralogy; transposition of the great arteries; PDA with reversal of shunt/Eisenmenger's syndrome [→ differential cyanosis]; tricuspid atresia; Ebstein's anomaly; pulmonary AV fistula).
  c Haemoglobin abnormalities:
    i Methaemoglobinaemia (congenital; acquired – drugs like nitrates and sulfonamides).
    ii Sulphaemoglobinaemia (drugs like nitrates and sulfonamides).
    iii Hb M disease.
    iv NADH diaphorase.

Signs of dehydration:
1 ↓ skin elasticity.
2 Rapid, low-volume (thready) pulse.
3 ↓ BP (postural or persistent hypotension).
4 Sunken eyes.
5 Dry tongue.
6 ↓ urine output.

Koilonychia:
1 Iron-deficiency anaemia.
2 Rarely d/t IHD/syphilis.

Onycholysis:
1 Psoriasis.
2 Hyperthyroidism.

Beau's lines (transverse furrows):
1 Any severe illness.

Onychomadesis (shedding of nail):
1 Any severe illness.

Longitudinal lines:
1 Lichen planus.
2 Alopecia areata.
3 Darier's disease.

Muehrcke's lines (white-coloured paired parallel transverse bands):
1 Hypoalbuminaemia.

---

2 Undersurface of lips, tongue and buccal mucosa *also* would be cold and bluish.

Mee's lines (single, white transverse band):
1 Organ failure (heart/renal).
2 Hodgkin's lymphoma.
3 Arsenic poisoning.

Nail pitting:
1 Psoriasis.
2 Alopecia areata.

Yellow nails:
1 Bronchiectasis.
2 Hypoalbuminaemia.
3 Lymphoedema.

Terry's nails (nail tips having dark pink or brown bands):
1 Old age (>75 yr).
2 CCF.
3 Cirrhosis of liver.
4 DM.
5 Malignancy.

Nail fold infarcts (d/t vasculitis) – dark blue-black areas in the nail folds:
1 SLE.
2 Subacute bacterial endocarditis (Osler's nodes).

Hand arthropathy (IP joints involved):
1 OA (DIP joints involved – Heberden's nodes).
2 RA (multiple abnormalities seen).
3 Psoriatic arthropathy (DIP or all IP joints involved).
4 SLE (DIP or all IP joints involved).

Hand and upper limb rashes:
1 Contact dermatitis.
2 Lichen planus.
3 Atopic eczema.
4 Psoriasis.

Pigmented creases, flexures and buccal mucosa – suggests ↑ ACTH:
1 Addison's disease.
2 Pituitary-driven Cushing's disease.
3 Ectopic ACTH secretion (from lung or other malignancy).

Swellings around the elbow joint:
1 OA.

  2 RA (rheumatoid nodules).
  3 Gouty tophi.
  4 Xanthomatosis (pale subcutaneous plaques attached to the underlying tendons).
  5 Limited range of neck movement, without stiffness: chronic cervical spondylosis with osteophytes.

Neck stiffness throughout the range of movement:
  1 Meningism (d/t viral/bacterial/tuberculous meningitis; SAH).
  2 Acute cervical spondylitis.
  3 Posterior fossa tumour.
  4 Anxiety (voluntary/semivoluntary resistance to movements).

Hair loss in a specific area:
  1 Alopecia areata/totalis.
  2 PCOS.
  3 Testosterone-secreting ovarian tumour.

Diffuse hair loss:
  1 Alopecia universalis.
  2 Any severe illness.
  3 Iron-deficiency anaemia.
  4 Pregnancy.
  5 Hypogonadism.
  6 Cytotoxic drugs.

Striking facial appearance:
  1 CNS pathology (parkinsonism; Huntington's chorea; bilateral UMN lesion d/t MND, myasthenia gravis, cerebrovascular disease).
  2 Endocrine pathology (acromegaly; hyper- or hypothyroidism; Cushing's syndrome).

Possible hypothermia (temp <35°C/95°F) – confirm with low-reading rectal thermometer:
  1 Prolonged exposure to cold weather/immersion.
  2 Hypothyroidism.

Arm span is more than double the sitting height:
  1 Marfan's syndrome.
  2 Hypogonadism.

Short limbs with normal trunk (sitting height is more than the length of the legs):
  1 Achondroplasia.

Limbs and trunk are proportionate but total height is below normal:
  1 Congenital hypopituitarism (pituitary dwarf).

Short 4th metacarpal (evident on making a fist) in a female:
  1 Turner's syndrome.

Short 4th/5th metacarpal:
  1 Pseudohypoparathyroidism.

Dactylitis:
  1 Sickle-cell anaemia.
  2 Sarcoidosis.
  3 Infection (TB; syphilis; sepsis).

Large and broad hands:
  1 Acromegaly.

Splinter haemorrhages:
  1 Normally seen in manual workers.
  2 Infective endocarditis.

Dark/black lesion below the nail plate:
  1 Splinter haemorrhage.
  2 Subungual haemorrhage.
  3 Subungual melanoma.

Leuconychia (white patches in nail plates):
  1 Seen in normal persons.
  2 Hypoalbuminaemia.

Osler's nodes (swellings in the pulps of terminal phalanges):
  1 Infective endocarditis (d/t vasculitis).

Heberden's nodes (osteophytes involving DIP joints):
  1 OA.

Bouchard's nodes (osteophytes involving PIP joints):
  1 OA.

Arachnodactyly (long and thin fingers):
  1 Marfan's syndrome.

Palmar erythema (redness of thenar and hypothenar eminences):
  1 Normal.

2 RA.
3 Thyrotoxicosis.
4 Liver disease.
5 Pregnancy.
6 OCPs.

Excessive palmar sweating:
1 Idiopathic.
2 Anxiety (palm is cold).
3 Thyrotoxicosis (palm is warm).

Puffiness of face:
1 Periorbital oedema (renal failure; acute glomerulonephritis → nephritic syndrome; nephrotic syndrome).
2 Myxoedema.
3 Angioedema.
4 Right heart failure (uncommonly and only when patient lies flat).

Redness of the cheeks (malar flush):
1 Normal.
2 Polycythaemia.
3 SLE.
4 Mitral stenosis.
5 Cushing's syndrome.

Xanthelasma:
1 Hyperlipidaemia.
2 Old age (even with normal lipid levels).

Subconjunctival haemorrhage:
1 Idiopathic.
2 Trauma.
3 Bleeding disorder.

Destruction of the nasal septum:
1 Wegener's granulomatosis.
2 Congenital syphilis.

Hyperpyrexia (rectal temperature ≥41°C/>106°F):
1 Heat stroke.
2 Malignant hyperpyrexia.
3 Neuroleptic malignant syndrome.
4 Pontine haemorrhage.
5 Thyrotoxic crisis.

6 Infection (malaria; septicaemia; viral infection).

7 Recreational drugs (amphetamines; cocaine).

Tongue enlargement:

1 Amyloidosis.

2 Acromegaly.

3 Thyroid pathology (myxoedema; cretinism).

Parotid swelling:

1 Parotid duct obstruction (d/t stone).

2 Parotid infection (suppurative parotitis; non-suppurative parotitis from ascending infection along parotid duct; mumps).

3 Parotid tumour.

4 Autoimmune disease (Sjögren's syndrome; sarcoidosis).

Lump in the face:

1 Parotid swelling.

2 Preauricular lymph node enlargement (infective/malignant).

3 Abscess/cyst (subcutaneous abscess; dental abscess; sebaceous cyst).

4 Malignancy (preauricular lymphoma; squamous/basal cell ca.; skin melanoma).

Hirsutism in female (hirsute upper lip, sideburns and chin; upwards extension of pubic hair):

1 Racial.

2 Ovarian pathology (PCOS; ovarian ca.).

3 Adrenal pathology (Cushing's syndrome; adrenal ca.).

4 Drugs (androgen analogues like Danazol, androgenic progestogens; phenytoin).

Hypertrichosis:

1 Hypothyroidism.

2 Malnutrition.

3 Porphyria.

4 Underlying malignancy (Hodgkin's lymphoma).

5 Drug-induced (minoxidil; corticosteroids; cyclosporin; penicillamine).

Submandibular lump (no movement with tongue protrusion or swallowing):
Submandibular gland enlargement:

1 Submandibular duct obstruction (d/t stone).

2 Submandibular infection (suppurative sialitis; non-suppurative sialitis from ascending infection along submandibular duct; mumps).

3 Submandibular tumour (adenocarcinoma; squamous cell ca., etc).

4 Autoimmune disease (Sjögren's syndrome; sarcoidosis).

Swellings other than submandibular gland:
1 Submandibular lymph node enlargement (infective/malignant).
2 Ranula (transilluminable cyst lateral to midline with domed bluish discolouration in the floor of mouth lateral to frenulum).
3 Submental dermoid (midline cyst in a <20-yr-old).

Anterior neck lump moving with tongue protrusion and swallowing (suggests extrathyroid lesion):
1 Thyroglossal cyst.
2 Ectopic thyroid tissue.

Neck lump moving with swallowing but not with tongue protrusion:
1 Goitre (euthyroid goitre; hypothyroid goitre; thyrotoxic goitre).

Goitre:
1 Sporadic.
2 Endemic (iodine deficiency).
3 Pregnancy.
4 Autoimmune thyroid disease.
5 Thyroiditis.
6 Drug-induced (ATDs;[3] lithium; amiodarone).

Euthyroid goitre:
1 Simple goitre.
2 Hashimoto's thyroiditis (euthyroid or hypothyroid).
3 Non-toxic MNG.
4 Thyroid enzyme deficiency – rare (euthyroid or hypothyroid).

Hypothyroid goitre:
1 Hashimoto's thyroiditis (euthyroid or hypothyroid).
2 Thyroid enzyme deficiency – rare (euthyroid or hypothyroid).

Hyperthyroid goitre:
1 Graves' disease.
2 Toxic MNG.
3 Toxic adenoma.

Solitary thyroid nodule:
1 Cyst (clinically euthyroid).
2 Adenoma (toxic/non-toxic).
3 Ca. (clinically euthyroid).

---

3   ATDs: antithyroid drugs.

Lump in anterior triangle (below digastric and in front of sternomastoid muscles):

1 Lymph node enlargement (infective; malignant [Hodgkin's or non-Hodgkin's lymphoma]).
2 Abscess (acute abscess; tuberculous 'cold' abscess).
3 Branchial cyst.
4 Cystic hygroma.
5 Carotid body tumour (chemodectoma).
6 Pharyngeal pouch.

Lump in posterior triangle (between sternomastoid and trapezius muscles):

1 Lymph node enlargement (infective/malignant [Hodgkin's or non-Hodgkin's lymphoma; metastases]).
2 Abscess (acute abscess; tuberculous 'cold' abscess).
3 Cystic hygroma.

Supraclavicular lump/s:

1 Lymph node enlargement (infective/malignant [Hodgkin's or non-Hodgkin's lymphoma; metastases from stomach or lungs]).
2 Subclavian artery aneurysm.

Axillary lymphadenopathy:

1 Lymph node enlargement (infective, e.g. viral prodrome, HIV infection, etc; malignant [reticulosis or primary tumour, metastases from ca. breast]).
2 Drugs (phenytoin; retroviral drugs).

Spider naevi:

1 In normal women (increased during periods).
2 OCPs.
3 Pregnancy.
4 Liver failure.

Early signs of PVD:

1 Shiny skin with loss of hair.

Pallor:

1 Anaemia.
2 Vasoconstriction (d/t shock, exposure to cold/Raynaud's phenomenon).

Subcutaneous emphysema:

1 Damage to the air-containing viscera (lungs; potentially pneumothorax, trachea; oesophagus).
2 Gas gangrene.

Campbell de Morgan's spots:
1 Commonly develop on the chest and abdomen with advancing age (red, 1–2 mm in diameter and don't blanch on pressure).

Erythema marginatum:
1 Rheumatic fever.

Galactorrhoea:
1 Pregnancy.
2 Prolactinoma.
3 Hypothyroidism.
4 Drugs (metoclopramide; domperidone; chlorpromazine and other tranquillisers).
5 Idiopathic.

Nipple abnormality:
1 Paget's disease of nipple with underlying malignancy.
2 Chronic infection → duct ectasia.
3 Duct papilloma.
4 Mamillary fistula (→ discharge from para-areolar region).

Breast lump/s:
1 Acute/chronic abscess.
2 Fat necrosis.
3 Cyst.
4 Fibroadenoma.
5 Benign fibrous mammary dysplasia.
6 Ca. (infiltrating ductal ca. or invasive lobar ca.).

Gynaecomastia:
1 Obesity.
2 Testicular problem (immature testes; primary or secondary hypogonadism; testicular tumour).
3 Chromosomal problem (Klinefelter's syndrome).
4 Cirrhosis of liver.
5 Ca. lung.
6 Drugs (digoxin; spironolactone; high alcohol intake).

Pressure sores:
1 Bedridden patient (d/t CVA; spinal cord injury, etc).
2 Poor nutrition.

Prominent leg veins (with or without leg swelling):
1 Varicose veins.

2 Thrombophlebitis.

3 DVT.

Unilateral ankle/calf oedema:

1 DVT/post-DVT venous insufficiency.

2 Cellulitis (from infection – primary, or secondary to insect bites).

3 Compression of large vein by tumour or lymph nodes.

4 Lymphatic obstruction/lymphoedema (infection, e.g. streptococcal lymphangitis [→ acute lymphatic obstruction]; filariasis/trypanosomiasis in tropics; malignant infiltration; Milroy's disease [congenital condition] – oedema present since childhood).

5 Ruptured Baker's cyst (leg swelling within seconds, usually while walking up a step; h/o arthritic knee usually present).

6 Immobility.

Common causes of bilateral ankle oedema:

1 CCF/cor pulmonale.

2 Hypoalbuminaemia d/t liver/renal disease; malnutrition, malabsorption or protein-losing enteropathy.

3 Poor venous return (d/t abdominal or pelvic masses, venous damage – postphlebitic or thrombotic).

4 Arterial/venous/lymphatic pathology (e.g. bilateral varicose veins/DVT; IVC obstruction; impaired lymphatic drainage).

5 Bilateral cellulitis.

6 Immobility.

Less-common causes of bilateral ankle oedema:

1 Pregnancy.

2 Immobility → dependent oedema.

3 Drugs (Ca^{2+} channel blockers, NSAIDs).

4 Wet beriberi (rare in western societies but commoner in Africa).

5 Idiopathic/cyclical oedema syndrome.

Pitting oedema (mechanism: ↑ interstitial fluid):

Generalised/bilateral:

1 Congestion (right heart failure; constrictive pericarditis; pericardial effusion; IVC/SVC obstruction).

2 Hypoproteinaemia (malnutrition; malabsorption; protein-losing enteropathy; cirrhosis of liver [→ ↓ protein synthesis]; nephrotic syndrome [→ ↑ protein loss]).

3 Pre-eclampsia.

Localised/unilateral:

1 Infection (e.g. cellulitis).

  2 Vascular causes (venous obstruction; angioedema).

  3 Immobile bedridden patient (d/t paralysis, etc).

Non-pitting oedema (mechanism: cutaneous deposition of some substance):

  1 Myxoedema (deposition of mucopolysaccharide).

  2 Angioedema ($\uparrow$ capillary permeability $\rightarrow$ leakage and deposition of plasma proteins).

  3 Lymphoedema (defective lymphatic drainage):

    a Lymphatic obstruction (infiltration by malignant cells; filariasis).

    b Iatrogenic (lymphadenectomy; irradiation of lymph nodes).

    c Congenital obstruction of lymphatics (Milroy's syndrome).

IVC obstruction:

  1 Exogenous compression (large ascites; ovarian cyst; enlarged para-aortic lymph nodes).

  2 Luminal obstruction (thrombosis).

SVC obstruction:

  1 Exogenous compression/infiltration:

    a Malignant lesion of the mediastinum (ca. lung; lymphoma; metastases).

    b Benign lesion of the mediastinum (retrosternal thyroid; thymoma; cyst [dermoid/hydatid]; aortic aneurysm).

  2 Luminal obstruction (thrombosis).

2 Cardiology

Tachycardia:
1 Physiologic (exercise; anxiety).
2 Anaemia.
3 Fever.
4 Thyroid problem (thyrotoxicosis).
5 Heart problem (tachyarrhythmias, e.g. SVT; IHD/MI; heart failure; hypotension/hypovolaemia; drugs like adrenaline, atropine, salbutamol, caffeine, alcohol, amphetamines).
6 Lung problem (hypoxia d/t any cause, e.g. pulmonary embolism).

Bradycardia:
1 Physiologic (athletes).
2 ↑ ICP.
3 Hypothermia.
4 Thyroid problem (hypothyroidism).
5 Heart problem (sick-sinus syndrome; complete heart block; drugs like digoxin, β-blockers – including eye drops; IHD/MI).
6 Obstructive jaundice.
7 Uraemia; electrolyte abnormalities.

Relative bradycardia:
1 Bacterial infections (enteric fever; meningitis with ↑ ICP).
2 Viral infections.

Sinus arrhythmia[1] (HR faster during inspiration; slower during expiration):
1 Physiologic.

Occasional premature beats:
1 Physiologic.

(Frequent premature beats in a heart patient may be pathologic).

Regularly irregular beats:
1 Digoxin toxicity (ventricular bigeminy/trigeminy).

---

1   Disappears in heart failure and autonomic neuropathy.

Irregularly irregular beats:
1 AF.
2 Atrial flutter with variable heart block (secondary to IHD, etc).
3 Frequent premature beats (secondary to IHD, etc).
4 Wenckebach heart block (secondary to IHD, etc).

Pulse deficit (difference between pulse rate and heart rate – counted by auscultation):
1 AF.

Slow-rising pulse (pulsus plateau):
1 AS (narrow pulse pressure).

Collapsing pulse (water-hammer pulse):
1 AR (wide pulse pressure).
2 VSD.
3 PDA.
4 Severe anaemia.

Pulsus bisferiens (two systolic peaks are palpable in one pulse; normal is one):
1 Combined AS and AR.

Jerky pulse:
1 HOCM.

Pulsus paradoxus (pulse becomes weak or impalpable during inspiration):
1 Pericardial pathology (massive pericardial effusion/cardiac tamponade; constrictive pericarditis).
2 Acute severe bronchial asthma (pulse pressure remains unchanged; in cardiac tamponade, it is reduced).

Pulsus alternans (a strong beat alternates with a weak beat and the beat-to-beat interval remains constant):
1 LVF.
2 SVT.

Pulsus bigeminus (a strong normal beat alternates with a weak premature beat; strong and weak beats occur close together and are followed by a long pause before the next pair):
1 Digoxin toxicity.

Radio–femoral delay:
1 Coarctation of aorta.

Low-volume pulse:
1 AS.
2 Heart failure (d/t any cause).
3 Hypovolaemic shock.
4 Septic shock ($\rightarrow$ poor vascular tone $\rightarrow$ low-volume pulse).

High-volume pulse:
1 Fever.
2 Severe anaemia.
3 Bradycardia (d/t any reason) with normal myocardium.
4 AR.
5 Hyperkinetic circulation (d/t fever; AV fistula; hypercapnia; thyrotoxicosis; Paget's disease).

Absent radial pulse:
1 Aortic dissection with subclavian involvement.
2 Trauma/surgery/catheterisation.
3 Arterial embolism.
4 Takayasu's arteritis.

Aortic dissection – predisposing conditions:
1 Essential HTN (in patients of Afro-Caribbean origin); secondary HTN (d/t coarctation of aorta).
2 Marfan's syndrome.
3 Ehlers–Danlos' syndrome.
4 Pregnancy.
5 Relapsing polychondritis.

Secondary hypertension:
1 Vascular hypertension (coarctation of aorta; subclavian artery stenosis).
2 Renal disease (glomerulonephritis; pyelonephritis; renal artery stenosis; ADPKD[2]).
3 Endocrine hypertension (Cushing's syndrome; Conn's syndrome/primary hyperaldosteronism; phaeochromocytoma; acromegaly).
4 OCPs; pregnancy (pre-eclampsia).
5 Neurogenic hypertension (post head injury; post stroke).
6 Drugs (OCPs – oestrogen containing; steroids; NSAIDs; erythropoietin).

Low blood pressure:
1 Cardiogenic shock.
2 Hypovolaemic shock.

---

2 USG criteria for ADPKD: age <30 yr – at least two cysts (unilateral or bilateral); 30–60 yr – at least two cysts in each kidney; >60 yr – at least four cysts in each kidney.

3 Loss of vascular tone (d/t septicaemia; adrenal failure, etc).

Postural hypotension (supine and standing BP after 1 minute – >10 mmHg fall; may be accompanied by dizziness):
1 Idiopathic (especially in elderly).
2 Autonomic neuropathy (d/t DM; tabes dorsalis – rarely).
3 Drugs: (high dose of antihypertensives; antidepressants; antipsychotics [phenothiazines]; antiparkinsonian drugs [L-dopa; carbidopa]).

BP/pulse difference between arms (R > L by 15 mmHg):
1 Aortic pathology (congenital supravalvular aortic stenosis; dissection of ascending aorta; aortic-arch syndrome/Takayasu's syndrome).
2 Subclavian steal syndrome.
3 Thoracic inlet syndrome.
4 Old or new thrombosis in an already atheromatous artery/aneurysm (complication of PVD).

BP/pulse difference between arm and legs (R > L by 15 mmHg) – wide cuff needed for thigh; arm and leg must be at same level:
1 Coarctation of aorta.
2 Dissection of descending thoracic aorta, abdominal aorta, iliac arteries (especially in a diabetic).
3 Old or new thrombosis in an already atheromatous artery/aneurysm (complication of PVD).

JVP:
1 **a wave:** right atrial contraction – end of atrial systole.
2 **x descent:** right atrial relaxation – beginning of atrial diastole.
3 **v wave:** right atrial filling – end of atrial diastole.
4 **y descent:** right atrial emptying – beginning of right ventricular diastole.

c wave is thought to be artefact seen on **x descent** (right atrial relaxation – beginning of atrial diastole) d/t carotid pulsations.

Prominent 'a' wave:
1 Right atrial and ventricular hypertrophy (d/t pulmonary hypertension; PS; TR).

Strikingly large 'a' waves (cannon waves) – seen when right atrium contracts against closed tricuspid valve:
1 Complete heart block.
2 Ventricular pacing with intact retrograde conduction.

Absent 'a' wave:
1 AF.

Prominent and palpable systolic wave on JVP:
1 TR (called ventricularisation of venous pulse).

Rapid 'y' descent:
1 Constrictive pericarditis.

Raised JVP:
1 Fluid overload.
2 Right heart failure:
   a Secondary to left heart failure.
   b Cor pulmonale.[3]
   c IHD.
   d Valvular/septal heart disease (PS; TS; TR; ASD).
   e Cardiomyopathy.
3 Arrhythmia (AF; complete heart block).
4 Pericardial disease (pericardial effusion; constrictive pericarditis).
5 Jugular vein obstruction.

Kussmaul's sign:
1 Constrictive pericarditis.
2 Tricuspid stenosis.
3 Right ventricular infarction.
4 Restrictive cardiomyopathy.

Pulsations along the parasternal border:
1 Right ventricular hypertrophy.

Pulsations in the left 2nd ICS:
1 Dilatation of the pulmonary artery.

Pulsations in the right 2nd ICS:
1 Aortic aneurysm.

Pulsations in the suprasternal notch:
1 AR.

Pulsations in the epigastrium:
1 Physiologic in thin individuals (d/t aorta).
2 AAA.

---

3   D/t: COPD; interstitial lung disease; recurrent pulmonary embolism; kyphoscoliosis.

3 Pulsatile liver (d/t TR).
4 Right ventricular hypertrophy.

Whole of the precordium moves with each cardiac beat:
1 Heart is greatly enlarged.

Apex beat shift:
Cardiac causes:
1 Hypertension.
2 IHD.
3 Valvular pathology (MR; AS; AR; VSD).
4 Dilated cardiomyopathy.
5 Occasionally d/t a grossly dilated right ventricle.

Non-cardiac causes:
1 Position of the patient (left lateral or sitting forward).
2 Chest deformity.
3 Pleural/pulmonary pathology causing mediastinal push/pull.

Impalpable apex beat:
1 Obesity/thick chest wall.
2 Lung pathology: emphysema.
3 Pericardial pathology: pericardial effusion.
4 Dextrocardia (apex beat palpable on the right side).

Tapping apex beat (beat is forceful but the palpating finger is not displaced):
1 Palpable loud 1st heart sound d/t MS.

Heaving apex beat (palpating finger is lifted):
Ill-sustained heave (occurs when left ventricle has to eject large blood volume):
1 MR.
2 AR.
3 VSD.

In all these conditions, left ventricle is enlarged. Thus apex beat is always displaced, as well as heaving.

Well-sustained heave (occurs when the left ventricle has to contract against high resistance):
1 AS.
2 Hypertension.

In both these conditions, left ventricle is hypertrophied initially but not enlarged. Thus apex beat, though heaving, is not displaced.

Apex beat displaced and heaving:
1 MR.
2 AR.
3 VSD.

Apex beat not displaced but heaving:
1 AS.
2 Hypertension.

Left parasternal heave (d/t right ventricular enlargement):
1 Pulmonary hypertension (which in turn could be d/t MS/MR; COPD, CRAD; primary pulmonary hypertension; kyphoscoliosis; longstanding ASD, VSD, PDA).
2 PS.
3 Fallot's tetralogy.

Palpable 1st heart sound (called tapping apex beat):
1 MS.

Palpable P_2:
1 Pulmonary hypertension.

Palpable A_2:
1 Systemic hypertension.

Palpable thrill in the neck (carotid shudder):
1 AS.

Loud S_1:
1 Tachycardia.
2 MS.

Soft S_1:
1 MR.
2 Heart failure.
3 Rheumatic carditis.

Variable intensity of S_1:
1 AF.
2 Complete heart block.

Loud P$_2$:
1 Pulmonary hypertension.

Soft P$_2$:
1 PS.

Loud A$_2$:
1 Systemic hypertension.

Soft A$_2$:
1 AS.
2 AR.

Both S$_1$ and S$_2$ are soft:
1 Thick chest wall.
2 Lung pathology: emphysema.
3 Pericardial pathology: pericardial effusion.

Splitting of S$_1$:
1 Arrhythmia (RBBB; LBBB; VT).
2 Valvular/septal defect (ASD; TS).

Splitting of S$_2$:
Usual splitting (A$_2$–P$_2$ interval is more during inspiration than expiration):
1 Physiologic (in children and young adults).
2 Pulmonary hypertension (split is narrow).
3 PS.
4 Dilated right ventricle.
5 RBBB.

Fixed splitting (A$_2$–P$_2$ interval is constant and wide):
1 ASD.

Reverse splitting (A$_2$–P$_2$ interval is less during inspiration than expiration):
1 Severe AS.
2 HOCM
3 LBBB.

S$_3$:
1 Physiologic (in children and young adults).
2 Pathological:[4]

---

4   D/t rapid ventricular filling.

    a   MR.
    b   Heart failure.
    c   Cardiomyopathy.
    d   Constrictive pericarditis.
    e   Hyperdynamic states (e.g. thyrotoxicosis; pregnancy).

S$_4$:
1   Physiologic (in children and young adults).
2   Pathological:[5]
    a   Left ventricular hypertrophy (d/t hypertension, HOCM).
    b   IHD (following MI → scarring of the infarcted tissue).
    c   Amyloid heart disease.

Gallop rhythm (S$_3$ + S$_4$):
1   Severe heart failure.

Heart failure → S$_3$; severe heart failure → gallop rhythm (S$_3$ + S$_4$).

Pericardial knock:
1   Pericardial pathology (constrictive pericarditis).

Opening snap after S$_2$ medial to the apex:
1   MS (it means that the valve cusps are stenosed but mobile).

Ejection systolic clicks soon after S$_1$:
Aortic click (at A$_1$ area and apex not affected by respiration):
1   AS.
2   Bicuspid aortic valve.

Pulmonary click (at pulmonary area and increases in intensity during expiration):
1   PS.
2   Dilatation of pulmonary artery (secondary to pulmonary hypertension or idiopathic).

Mid-systolic click:
1   MVP.

Systolic murmurs:
Pansystolic:
1   MR.

---

5   D/t the increased atrial contraction required to fill a stiff left ventricle. It doesn't occur in AF.

  2 TR.
  3 MR + TR.
  4 VSD.

Ejection systolic:
  1 AS.
  2 Aortic sclerosis.
  3 HOCM.[6]
  4 PS.
  5 Pulmonary high flow (e.g. d/t ASD).

Diastolic murmurs:
Mid-diastolic:
  1 MS.
  2 MS with pliable valve (suggested by opening snap).
  3 TS.
  4 ASD (flow murmur at tricuspid area).
  5 PDA (flow murmur at mitral area).
  6 AR (heard at apex – called Austin Flint's murmur). It occurs d/t the movement of anterior mitral leaflet between two streams of blood – one from the left atrium and other from the aorta. It is differentiated from MS on the basis of S_1 – not loud, and opening snap – absent.
  7 Acute rheumatic carditis (heard at apex – called Carey Coombs' murmur).

Early diastolic:
  1 AR.
  2 PR.
  3 Pulmonary hypertension ($\rightarrow$ functional pulmonary regurgitation – called Graham Steell's murmur).

Continuous 'machinery' murmur (systolic + diastolic):
  1 PDA.
  2 Mixed aortic valve disease.
  3 Pericardial rub (scratching murmur).
  4 Venous hum (positional).

Systolic murmur at tricuspid area:
  1 TS.
  2 VSD.
  3 HOCM.

---

6   Increased by Valsalva manoeuvre.

Systolic murmur at mitral area:
1 MR (↑ intensity on squatting; ↓ on standing and Valsalva manoeuvre).
2 MVP.
3 HOCM.

In both MVP and HOCM, the intensity is less when patient is in squatting position; however, it increases on standing and with Valsalva manoeuvre.

ASD (congenital) + MS (acquired) = Lutembacher's syndrome.

MS:
1 Rheumatic fever.

MR:
1 Rheumatic fever.
2 IHD (infarction → rupture of papillary muscle).
3 Left ventricular dilatation (→ dilatation of mitral valve ring).

TR:
1 Right ventricular dilatation.

AS:
Valvular stenosis:
1 >65-yr-old: degenerative changes and calcification in a congenitally bicuspid valve.
2 40–50-yr-old: congenital AS.
3 Rheumatic fever (uncommonly).

Subvalvular stenosis:
1 Congenital web.
2 HOCM.

Supravalvular aortic stenosis:
1 Congenital.
2 Coarctation of aorta.
3 Williams' syndrome.

AR:
1 Infection (rheumatic fever; infective endocarditis).
2 Congenital (bicuspid valve; Marfan's syndrome).

PS:
1 Congenital.
2 Carcinoid syndrome (a late sign).

PR:
1 Pulmonary hypertension (→ dilatation of pulmonary ring → early diastolic murmur – called Graham Steell's murmur).

Signs of mitral stenosis (MS):
1 Pulse may be irregularly irregular (d/t AF).
2 Tapping apex beat.
3 Diastolic thrill at apex.
4 Loud S_1.
5 Opening snap (best audible medial to the apex).
6 Mid-diastolic murmur (low-pitched, rough, rumbling in character with presystolic accentuation; best heard at apex in left lateral position with the bell).

Complications of MS:
1 Left atrial (AF; thromboembolism [→ stroke]; infective endocarditis[7]).
2 Pulmonary (acute pulmonary oedema; pulmonary hypertension [→ right heart failure]; haemoptysis).
3 Oesophageal (dysphagia [enlarged left atrium → oesophageal compression]).
4 Left recurrent laryngeal nerve (hoarseness of voice d/t nerve compression).

Signs of mitral regurgitation (MR):
1 Pulse is high volume.
2 Apex beat shifted to the left.
3 Ill-sustained heave.
4 Systolic thrill at the apex.
5 Soft S_1.
6 Pansystolic murmur at the apex radiating to the axilla; louder during expiration.

Signs of tricuspid regurgitation (TR):
1 Large systolic wave in the JVP.
2 Pulsatile liver.
3 Right ventricular heave.
4 Pansystolic murmur with maximum intensity at the tricuspid area; louder during inspiration.

Signs of atrial stenosis (AS):
1 Slow-rising pulse; pulse pressure is narrow.
2 Apex beat remains undisplaced except in the very advanced cases; well-sustained heave.
3 Systolic thrill at the aortic area.

---

7   Uncommon in pure MS.

4 Carotid shudder.
5 Soft A_2.
6 Systolic click (if AS is at the valvular level).
7 Ejection systolic murmur with maximum intensity at the aortic area radiating to the neck; louder during expiration.

Signs of aortic regurgitation (AR):
1 Collapsing pulse; wide pulse pressure; pistol shot sounds over femoral area.
2 Apex beat shifted with ill-sustained heave.
3 Soft A_2.
4 Early diastolic murmur with maximum intensity at the A_2 area (i.e. 3rd left ICS); best heard when patient leans forward and holds breath in expiration.

Signs of pulmonary stenosis (PS):
1 Right ventricular heave.
2 Systolic thrill at the pulmonary area.
3 Soft P_2.
4 Systolic click at the pulmonary may be heard.
5 Ejection systolic murmur with maximum intensity at the pulmonary area radiating to the left shoulder; louder during inspiration.

Signs of VSD:
1 Pulse is high volume.
2 Apex beat shifted to the left with ill-sustained heave.
3 Systolic thrill at left parasternal border.
4 Normal S_1.
5 Pansystolic murmur best audible at the 4th ICS to the left of the sternum; louder during expiration; doesn't radiate to the axilla; may, however, radiate across the sternum.

Signs of ASD:[8]
1 Left parasternal heave.
2 Wide and fixed splitting of S_2.
3 Ejection systolic murmur at pulmonary area.
4 Mid-diastolic flow murmur at tricuspid area.
5 ECG shows RV conduction delay; radiograph shows dilated pulmonary arteries and increased vascularity.
6 Echocardiography/Doppler is diagnostic.
7 A patent foramen ovale is present in 25% of the population; it can lead to paradoxic emboli and CVA.[9]

---

8   Often asymptomatic; usually diagnosed incidentally on routine physical examination.
9   It should be particularly suspected in patients who have cryptogenic stroke before age 55 yr.

Venous hum (continuous murmur-like sound audible in the neck when the patient is standing, sitting or reclining against pillow; disappears when patient assumes a horizontal or head-down position):
1 Kinking of large neck veins (common in children).

Eisenmenger's syndrome:[10]
1 ASD.
2 VSD.
3 PDA.

HOCM – signs:
1 Jerky pulse.
2 Prominent 'a' wave on JVP.
3 Forceful apex.
4 4th heart sound.
5 Ejection systolic murmur (increased on standing from a squatting position).

Chest pain:
1 Ischaemic heart disease (MI; angina pectoris).
2 Oesophageal disease (diffuse oesophageal spasm; reflux oesophagitis).
3 Serositis (pleuritis; pericarditis).
4 Pulmonary embolism.
5 Spontaneous pneumothorax.
6 Dissection of aorta.
7 Musculoskeletal chest pain.
8 Non-specific chest pain; precordial catch.
9 Diseases of the spine.
10 Herpes zoster.

Chest pain in a young female – emergencies:
1 Myocarditis.
2 Acute MI (if present rule out inherited lipid disorders or conditions that increase the risk of thrombosis, e.g. SLE or Behçet's syndrome).
3 Dissection of aorta (especially if has marfanoid features).
4 Pulmonary embolism.

Causes of retrosternal/central chest pain:
1 Cardiac disease (MI; angina pectoris; pericarditis).
2 Oesophageal disease (diffuse oesophageal spasm; reflux oesophagitis).
3 Tracheal disease (tracheitis).
4 Aortic disease (dissection).
5 Pulmonary embolism.

---

10 Develops when pulmonary hypertension causes reversal of blood flow.

6 Musculoskeletal chest pain.

Chest pain – aggravated by breathing or movement:
1 Serous membranes pathology (pleuritis; pneumothorax; pericarditis).
2 Lung pathology (pulmonary infarction).
3 Chest wall pathology (musculoskeletal injury; musculoskeletal inflammation, e.g. Bornholm's disease caused by Coxsackie B infection; Tietze's syndrome).
4 Nerve pathology (herpes zoster [shingles]; referred cervical root pain).

Severe lower chest or upper abdominal pain:
1 MI (often inferior wall).
2 Gastritis/GORD.
3 Pancreatitis (often d/t gallstone impaction in CBD).
4 Biliary colic.

Spine diseases that cause chest pain:
1 Trauma.
2 Tuberculosis of the spine.
3 Extradural tumours of the spinal cord.
4 Metastases.

Angina/MI with normal coronary arteries:
1 Muscle hypertrophy (HOCM; hypertensive heart disease; AS; AR).
2 Vasculopathy (coronary arteritis especially PAN; coronary artery embolus secondary to intramural thrombus or vegetation).
3 Pulmonary hypertension.
4 Severe anaemia.
5 Endocrinopathy (thyrotoxicosis; phaeochromocytoma).
6 Drug abuse (cocaine; amphetamines).

These causes should be particularly excluded when a young person presents with ischaemic chest pain.

Sudden death in a young elite athlete:
1 Cardiac causes:
   a Muscle pathology (HOCM [50%]; arrhythmogenic right ventricular cardiomyopathy; myocarditis).
   b Vasculopathy (coronary artery anomaly).
   c Valvular pathology (MVP).
   d WPW syndrome; LQTS.
   e Drug abuse.
2 Non-cardiac causes:
   a Rhabdomyolysis.

b Heat stroke.

c Sarcoidosis.

MI – early complications:

1 Arrhythmias:
   a Atrial/ventricular ectopics; sinus bradycardia; atrial tachycardia; AF; VT; VF.
   b Heart blocks – 1st, 2nd or 3rd degree (more common in cases of inferior wall MI).
   c LBBB; RBBB.
2 Cardiogenic shock.
3 Pulmonary oedema.
4 MR (d/t papillary muscle infarction and rupture).
5 VSD (d/t septal infarction and rupture).
6 Pericarditis; haemopericardium (d/t ventricular wall infarction and rupture → cardiac tamponade).
7 Thromboembolism.
8 Sudden death.

MI – late complications:

1 Recurrent arrhythmias.
2 Heart failure.
3 Dressler's syndrome.[11]
4 Ventricular aneurysm.

Myocarditis:

1 Infection (viral [e.g. Coxsackie; influenza]; bacterial [e.g. acute rheumatic fever; diphtheria]; protozoal [e.g. Chagas' disease; toxoplasmosis]; rickettsial).
2 Toxins (e.g. lead).
3 Drugs (e.g. chloroquine).
4 Peripartum.

Infective endocarditis – predisposing factors:

1 Valvular pathology (MS [secondary to rheumatic heart disease]; MVP; bicuspid aortic valve; prosthetic valve).
2 Hypertrophic cardiomyopathy.
3 IV drug abuse.

Culture-positive infective endocarditis – aetiological agents:

1 Common: *Streptococcus viridans*; *Staphylococcus aureus*.

---

11 It is an autoimmune reaction to necrotic myocardium occurring weeks to months after acute MI. It presents with fever, pericarditis and pleuritis.

2 Prosthetic valves:
  a Within 1 yr of surgery: *Staphylococcus aureus/epidermidis*.
  b After 1 yr of surgery: *Streptococcus viridans*; *Staphylococcus aureus*.
3 IV drug abuser: *Staphylococcus aureus*; gram-negative bacilli (less common).
4 Associated with ca. colon: *Streptococcus faecalis*.

Culture-negative endocarditis:
1 Infective:
  a *Brucella* spp.
  b *Chlamydia* spp.
  c *Coxiella burnetti*.
  d *Legionella* spp.
  e *Mycoplasma* spp.
  f *Tropheryma whippelii*.
  g Fungi/histoplasmosis.
2 Non-infective:
  a SLE (Libman–Sacks' endocarditis).
  b Marantic endocarditis.

Endocarditis from animals/birds – causative organisms:
1 Sheep/cattle: *Coxiella burnetti*.
2 Cats: *Bartonella henselae*.
3 Birds: *Chlamydophila psittaci*.

Complications of infective endocarditis:
1 Embolic phenomenon (stroke; MI; peripheral arterial; pulmonary).
2 Mycotic aneurysm.[12]
3 Rupture of cusp of a valve (→ sudden deterioration of heart failure).

Pericarditis (→ pericardial effusion/constrictive pericarditis):
1 Infection (TB; bacterial [e.g. staphylococcus]; viral [e.g. Coxsackie]).
2 MI (acute MI; post-MI syndrome/Dressler's syndrome).
3 Rheumatic fever.
4 Uraemia.
5 Connective tissue disorders.
6 Myxoedema.
7 Malignancy.

Pleuritis:
1 Infection (pneumonia; TB).
2 Connective tissue disorders.
3 Pulmonary infarction.

---

12 Infection of the wall of an artery d/t infective embolism leading to aneurysm formation.

4 Uraemia.

5 Malignancy (metastases; mesothelioma).

Acute dyspnoea:
1 Asthma attack.
2 Pneumonia.
3 Pulmonary oedema.[13]
4 Pulmonary embolism.
5 Pleural disease (spontaneous pneumothorax; massive pleural effusion).

Acute respiratory distress syndrome (ARDS):
1 Acute pancreatitis.
2 Aspiration of gastric contents.
3 Septicaemia.
4 Major trauma.

Metabolic acidosis:
1 Renal failure.
2 Diabetic ketoacidosis.
3 Lactic acidosis.
4 Salicylate, methanol or ethylene glycol poisoning.

Chronic dyspnoea:
1 Heart failure (LVF; RVF; CCF).
2 COPD (chronic bronchitis; emphysema).
3 Asthma.
4 Obesity.
5 Interstitial lung disease.
6 Severe anaemia.
7 Psychogenic.

Left heart failure:
1 HTN.
2 IHD.
3 Valvular/septal heart disease (MS; MR; AS; AR; VSD).
4 Cardiomyopathy.

Right heart failure:
1 Secondary to left heart failure.
2 Cor pulmonale.[14]
3 IHD.

---

13 D/t cardiac disease/LVF ($\uparrow$ PCWP) or non-cardiac disease – ARDS (normal PCWP).

14 D/t: COPD; interstitial lung disease; recurrent pulmonary embolism; kyphoscoliosis.

4 Valvular/septal heart disease (PS; TS; TR; ASD).
5 Cardiomyopathy.

Right heart failure with normal left heart:
1 Cor pulmonale.
2 Right ventricular infarction.
3 Valvular/septal heart disease (PS; TS; TR; ASD).

Precipitating factors for heart failure:
1 Physical over-exertion; excessive salt and water intake.
2 Anaemia.
3 Thyrotoxicosis.
4 Infections.
5 Heart pathologies (infective endocarditis; MI; arrhythmias).
6 Pulmonary embolism.
7 Pregnancy.

Complications of heart failure:
1 Uraemia.
2 Electrolyte disturbances ($\downarrow$ Na$^+$; $\downarrow$ K$^+$).
3 Liver impairment (congestive cirrhosis).
4 Arrhythmias (both atrial and ventricular).[15]
5 Thromboembolism (DVT/PE/systemic d/t AF or intracardiac thrombus).
6 Weight loss.

Simultaneous heart and renal failure:
1 HTN.
2 DM.
3 Generalised (coronary and renovascular) atherosclerosis.
4 Vasculitides (PAN, etc).
5 Thrombosis (antiphospholipid syndrome).
6 Emboli (infective endocarditis).
7 Fibrosis (systemic sclerosis; amyloidosis).
8 Ethylene glycol poisoning.

Congenital acyanotic heart diseases:
1 Left-to-right shunt:
  a ASD.
  b VSD.
  c PDA.
  d Coarctation of aorta with associated VSD or PDA.
2 Without a shunt:

---

15 Responsible for up to 50% of the deaths in patients with cardiac failure.

    a Congenital aortic stenosis.

    b Coarctation of aorta without associated VSD or PDA.

Congenital cyanotic heart diseases:

1 Right-to-left shunt:
   a Fallot's tetralogy.
   b Transposition of great vessels.
   c Severe Ebstein's anomaly.
2 Without a shunt:
   a Tricuspid atresia.
   b Severe pulmonary stenosis.
   c Pulmonary atresia.
   d Hypoplastic left heart.
3 Reversal of a previous left-to-right shunt (d/t ASD, VSD, PDA):
   a Eisenmenger's syndrome.

Patent ductus arteriosus (PDA):

1 Maternal rubella.

Coarctation of aorta – causes:

1 Congenital.
2 Rarely acquired (Takayasu's arteritis; trauma).

Coarctation of aorta – disease associations:

1 Heart-related (valvular pathologies, e.g. bicuspid aortic valve [50%]; MVP; VSD; PDA).
2 Renal abnormalities.
3 Berry aneurysms.
4 Turner's syndrome.

Drugs that cause hypertension:

1 Steroids (corticosteroids; mineralocorticoids; anabolic steroids).
2 Oestrogen-containing OCPs.
3 NSAIDs.
4 Sympathomimetics (ephedrine).

Pulmonary hypertension:

1 Valvular/septal diseases (MS; MR; ASD; VSD; PDA).
2 COPD.
3 Chronic restrictive airway disease.
4 Recurrent pulmonary emboli.
5 Kyphoscoliosis.
6 Primary.

Signs of pulmonary hypertension:
1 Prominent 'a' wave in JVP.
2 Palpable P_2.
3 Left parasternal heave.
4 Loud P_2.
5 Closely split S_2.
6 Graham-Steell's murmur.

DVT:
1 Prolonged bed rest (e.g. after surgery).
2 Pelvic infection.
3 Pelvic operation (orthopaedic; urological, etc).
4 OCPs.
5 CCF.
6 Long air travel.

Venous and arterial thromboses:
1 Paradoxical emboli.
2 Homocystinuria.
3 Sickle-cell anaemia.
4 Paroxysmal nocturnal haemoglobinuria.
5 Myeloproliferative disorders.

Fat embolism:
1 Blunt trauma (90%).
2 Acute pancreatitis.

Orthopnoea and PND:
1 Pulmonary oedema.
2 Asthma.
3 COPD.

Palpitations:
1 Rhythm disturbances (sinus tachycardia; runs of SVT; AF; episodic heart block; ventricular ectopics).
2 Endocrine pathology (thyrotoxicosis; phaeochromocytoma).
3 Menopause.

Diagnostic criteria of peripartum cardiomyopathy:
The following four criteria must be met:
1 Woman presenting with heart failure during the last month of pregnancy or within five months postpartum.
2 No obvious cause of heart failure found (peripartum cardiomyopathy is a diagnosis of exclusion).

3 Previously normal cardiac status.

4 Left ventricular systolic dysfunction on echocardiography.

Restrictive cardiomyopathy:

1 Endomyocardial fibrosis (EMF).

2 Systemic sclerosis.

3 Amyloidosis.

4 Haemochromatosis.

5 Carcinoid syndrome.

Side effects of amiodarone:

1 Ocular (corneal deposits [$\rightarrow$ glare of headlights at night – reversible when the drug is stopped]; photosensitivity; optic neuritis).

2 Nightmares.

3 Metallic taste.

4 Hyper- or hypothyroidism.

5 Arrhythmias (especially torsades de pointes).

6 Alveolitis/pulmonary fibrosis.

7 Hepatitis/cirrhosis.

8 Epididymitis.

9 Myopathy.

10 Peripheral neuropathy.

Digoxin toxicity – features:

1 Arrhythmias (especially AV block).

2 Nausea, vomiting, diarrhoea.

3 Headache; dizziness.

4 Seizures.

5 Xanthopsia (yellow vision).

6 Skin reactions.

7 Impotence.

Digoxin toxicity – causes:

1 Electrolyte disturbances ($\downarrow K^+$; $\downarrow Mg^{2+}$; $\uparrow Ca^{2+}$).

2 Renal impairment.

3 Hypothyroidism.

4 Drug-induced (ACEI;[16] Ca^{2+} channel blockers; amiodarone;[17] quinidine; cyclosporine).

Digoxin toxicity – management:

- Prevent absorption: gastric lavage; activated charcoal (if patient

---

16 ACEI reduce renal clearance of digoxin $\rightarrow$ digoxin toxicity.

17 Amiodarone displaces digoxin from the binding proteins $\rightarrow$ digoxin toxicity.

presents within 6–8 hr of ingestion).
- Correct electrolyte disturbances ($\downarrow$ K$^+$; $\downarrow$ Mg^{2+}; $\uparrow$ Ca^{2+}).
- For bradyarrhythmia: atropine; temporary pacemaker for symptomatic bradycardia that has failed to respond to atropine.
- For SVT: verapamil.
- For VT: lignocaine; phenytoin.

Digoxin toxicity – indications of digoxin-binding antibody fragment:[18]
1 Reserved for very severe cases alone, i.e.:
  a Patients who have taken a large overdose ($\geq$10 mg in adults and $\geq$4 mg in children).
  b Serum digoxin level >13 nmol/L.
  c Serum K$^+$ level >5 mmol/L.
  d Presence of life-threatening arrhythmias (2nd or 3rd degree AV block; VT; VF).

Contraindications to thrombolysis (list includes both absolute and relative contraindications):
1 Internal bleeding.
2 History of major trauma, head injury, recent surgery, or liver/kidney biopsy in the last two weeks.
3 Intracranial neoplasm; previous proven haemorrhagic CVA.[19]
4 Active diabetic proliferative retinopathy.
5 BP >200/120 mmHg.
6 Suspected aortic aneurysm/aortic dissection/intracardiac thrombus.
7 Bleeding disorder or patient on anticoagulant therapy with INR >1.8.
8 Pregnancy/postpartum/current menstrual bleeding.
9 Prolonged or traumatic CPR.

Absolute contraindication of thrombolysis:
1 Active bleeding.
2 Cerebral haemorrhage (ever).
3 Intracranial neoplasm.
4 Aortic dissection.

Primary hyperlipidaemia:
1 Familial hypercholesterolaemia.
2 Familial hypertriglyceridaemia.
3 Familial combined hyperlipidaemia.
4 Lipoprotein lipase deficiency ($\rightarrow$ failure to break down chylomicrons).

---

18 Normally given as IV infusion over 30 min. In cases of cardiac arrest, it can be given as IV bolus. It freely filters through the kidneys and thus can be given even in CRF patients.

19 Cerebral infarct within the last three months (controversial).

Secondary hyperlipidaemia:

1 Mainly hypercholesterolaemia:
   a Hypothyroidism.
   b Cholestasis (PBC; PSC).
   c Renal pathology (nephrotic syndrome; renal transplant).
   d Multiple myeloma.
2 Mainly hypertriglyceridaemia:
   a Obesity.
   b Chronic alcoholism.
   c Chronic liver disease.
   d Diabetes mellitus (insulin resistance).
   e Drugs (thiazides; high-dose oestrogen).

CXR – left ventricular failure:

1 Heart size enlarged (mainly to the left of midline) with central trachea.
2 Linear upper-lobe opacities (d/t venous dilatation).
3 Fluffy lung opacities centrally more than peripherally.

CXR – pulmonary hypertension:

1 Unusually convex right heart border.
2 Upwardly rounded apex.
3 Bilaterally prominent hilar shadows.

CXR – ASD:

1 Unusually convex right heart border.
2 Upwardly rounded apex.
3 Bilaterally prominent hilar shadows.

CXR – cardiomyopathy:

1 Heart size enlarged with clear borders (indicating poor contraction).[20]

CXR – pericardial effusion:

1 Large globular cardiac outline with clear borders (indicating poor contraction).

CXR – mitral stenosis:

1 Heart size may be enlarged.
2 Enlarged left atrium (shown as rounded opacity behind the heart which splays the carinal angle).
3 ± calcification in the position of mitral valve; ± dense nodules d/t haemosiderosis.

---

20 History of predisposing conditions like chronic alcoholism, RA, amyloidosis, leukaemia. Echo shows ↓ ejection fraction.

CXR – left ventricular aneurysm:
1 Bulge in the left ventricular border ± calcification (h/o IHD).

CXR – mediastinal emphysema:
1 Gas around the mediastinal contour (surgical emphysema may be found clinically).

CXR – hiatus hernia:
1 Circular shadow behind the heart ± air-fluid level.
2 Absent gastric air bubble.

3 ECG

Sinus rhythm – key ECG features:
1 Normal heart rate (60–100/min).
2 Upright P waves in lead II and inverted in lead aVR.
3 QRS complex after every P wave.

Heart rate:
1 300 large squares correspond to 1 minute.
2 30 large squares correspond to 6 seconds.

If heart rate is >100/min, consider:
1 Narrow-complex tachycardia.
2 Broad-complex tachycardia.

Narrow-complex (<3 small squares) tachycardia: always supraventricular in origin:
1 Sinus tachycardia.
2 Paroxysmal atrial/junctional tachycardia.
3 Atrial flutter/fibrillation.
4 AV re-entry tachycardia.

Sinus tachycardia – key ECG features:
1 Heart rate >100/min.
2 Upright P waves in lead II and inverted in lead aVR.
3 QRS complex after every P wave.

Sinus tachycardia:
1 Physiologic (exercise; anxiety).
2 Anaemia.
3 Fever.
4 Thyroid problem (thyrotoxicosis).
5 Heart problem (tachyarrhythmias, e.g. SVT, IHD/MI, heart failure; hypotension/hypovolaemia; drugs like adrenaline, atropine, salbutamol, caffeine, alcohol, amphetamines).
6 Lung problem (hypoxia d/t any cause, e.g. pulmonary embolism).

Broad-complex (>3 small squares) tachycardia: often ventricular in origin:
1 Narrow-complex tachycardia with aberrant conduction.
2 VT.

3 Accelerated idioventricular rhythm.

4 Torsades de pointes.

Clues that suggest a broad-complex tachycardia is VT (and not SVT):

1 VT is more common in an elderly patient with a history of cardiac disease, as opposed to a young patient with no previous history of cardiac disease, in whom SVT with aberrant conduction is more likely.

2 VT generally causes 'atypical' broad complexes that do not have the classic morphology of LBBB or RBBB. If typical LBBB or RBBB morphology is seen, SVT with aberrant conduction is more likely.

3 Fusion[1]/capture beats[2] (infrequent).

4 QRS complex characteristics:

    a A 1:1 relationship b/w P waves and QRS complexes usually means a supraventricular origin, except in the case of VT with retrograde conduction.

    b Monophasic (R) or biphasic (qR, QR or RS) complexes in V_1; and a qR or QS complex in V_6.[3]

    c Ventricular rate <170/min (higher rate favours SVT).

    d QRS duration 3.5 small squares (>0.14 sec). In SVT, it is >0.12 sec, but <0.14 sec.

    e QRS direction – same in leads V_1–V_6 – called concordance.

    f QRS axis: a shift in the axis of ≥40° (left or right); left axis deviation with right bundle branch block morphology.

5 No effect by adenosine.

If heart rate is <60/min, consider:

1 Sinus pathology:

    a Sinus bradycardia.

    b Sick-sinus syndrome.

    c Sinus arrest with consequent escape rhythms (AV junctional escape rhythm; ventricular escape rhythm).

2 AV nodal pathology:

    a 2nd or 3rd degree AV block.

3 Drug-induced bradycardia.

4 Asystole.

---

1   Fusion beat appears when the ventricles are activated by an atrial impulse, and a ventricular impulse generated by a ventricular focus discharges simultaneously.

2   In a rhythm strip showing broad-complex tachycardia, a capture beat develops when an atrial impulse manages to 'capture' the ventricles for a beat, causing a narrow QRS complex to appear, which may be preceded by a normal P wave.

3   A triphasic QRS complex in leads I and V_6 favours SVT.

Sinus bradycardia – key ECG features:
1 Heart rate <60/min.
2 Upright P waves in lead II and inverted in lead aVR.
3 QRS complex after every P wave.

Sinus bradycardia:
1 Physiologic (athletes).
2 ↑ ICP.
3 Hypothermia.
4 Thyroid problem (hypothyroidism).
5 Heart problem (sick-sinus syndrome; complete heart block; drugs like digoxin, β-blockers – including eye drops; IHD/MI).
6 Obstructive jaundice.
7 Uraemia; electrolyte abnormalities.

Sinus arrhythmia – key ECG features:
1 Every P wave is followed by a QRS complex.
2 Heart rate varies with respiration (inspiration → ↑ heart rate; expiration → ↓ heart rate).

Sick-sinus syndrome – causes:
1 Degeneration and fibrosis of the sinus node (commonest cause).
2 IHD.
3 Myocarditis/cardiomyopathy.
4 Amyloidosis.
5 Drugs (e.g. digoxin, β-blockers).

Arrhythmias in sick-sinus syndrome:
1 Sinus bradycardia/sinus arrest/SA block.
2 Atrial tachycardia/flutter/fibrillation.
3 AV nodal conduction disorders.

Sinus arrest – key ECG features:
1 On an ECG strip, a P wave will suddenly fail to appear at the expected place.
2 After a gap of variable length, an atrial (P wave of different shape) or junctional (P wave usually absent) escape beat is seen.

Sinus block – key ECG features:
1 On an ECG strip, a P wave will suddenly fail to appear at the expected place.
2 No escape beat is seen.
3 After a gap, next SA nodal beat (identical P wave) appears at the expected place.

Atrial escape rhythm – key ECG features:
1 Heart rate 60–80/min.
2 P waves are not identical to the previous P waves generated by the SA node.
3 Narrow QRS complex.

Junctional escape rhythm – key ECG features:
1 Heart rate 40–60/min.
2 Absent/inverted P waves.
3 Narrow QRS complex.

Ventricular escape rhythm – key ECG features:
1 Heart rate 20–40/min.
2 Absent P waves.
3 Broad QRS complex.

Atrial ectopic beat – key ECG features:
1 P wave earlier than expected.
2 P wave not identical to the previous P waves generated by the SA node.

AV junctional ectopic beat – key ECG features:
1 QRS complex earlier than expected.
2 Narrow QRS complex.

Ventricular ectopic beat – key ECG features:
1 QRS complex earlier than expected.
2 Broad QRS complex.

Atrial tachycardia – key ECG features:[4]
1 Heart rate >100/min (usually 150–250/min).
2 Abnormally shaped P waves (P waves generated by the atrial focus are different in morphology compared to those being generated by the SA node).[5]

AV re-entry tachycardia/AV nodal re-entry tachycardia – key ECG features:
1 Heart rate >100/min (usually 150–250/min).
2 P waves not seen (embedded in the QRS complexes) or inverted P waves seen.

---

4   Atrial tachycardia differs from sinus tachycardia in that the impulses are generated by an ectopic focus somewhere within the atrial myocardium, instead of SA node.

5   In both sinus and atrial tachycardia, at high rates the P wave may start to overlap with the T wave of the previous beat, making it hard to identify.

3 When visible, there is one P wave per QRS complex present.

4 QRS complexes are regular and narrow (unless some aberrant conduction is present).

Atrial tachycardia + AV block:[6]

1 Digoxin toxicity.

Paroxysmal atrial/junctional tachycardia:

1 Digoxin toxicity; tobacco; caffeine.

2 Sick-sinus syndrome.

3 WPW syndrome.

4 IHD.

5 MS.

6 Dilated cardiomyopathy.

7 Pulmonary pathology (COPD).

8 Endocrine pathology (thyrotoxicosis).

Atrial flutter or fibrillation (AF):

1 HTN.

2 IHD.

3 Valvular/septal pathology (MS; ASD).

4 Dilated cardiomyopathy.

5 Thyrotoxicosis.

6 Pericardial pathology (constrictive pericarditis).

7 Pulmonary pathology (pneumonia; pulmonary embolism).

Atrial flutter – key ECG features:

1 Atrial rate around 300/min (range = 250–350/min).

2 'Sawtooth' baseline.

3 AV block (most commonly 2:1 block; could be 3:1 or 4:1).

Atrial fibrillation – key ECG features:

1 Absent P waves.

2 Irregularly irregular QRS (ventricular) rhythm.

Indications of warfarin therapy in a case of AF:

(Given when the risk of thromboembolism is high.)

1 Age ≥75 yr.

2 MS.

3 ↓ LV ejection fraction (d/t IHD).

4 Uncontrolled HTN.

6　At atrial rates above 200/min, the AV node struggles to keep up with impulse conduction and AV block may occur.

5 Previous TIA or stroke.

Multifocal atrial tachycardia (MAT) – key ECG features:
1 P waves of variable shapes (d/t origin from different foci).
2 Irregularly irregular ventricular rhythm.
3 Ventricular rate >100/min.

Wandering pacemaker – key ECG features:
1 P waves of variable shapes (d/t origin from different foci).
2 Irregularly irregular ventricular rhythm.
3 Ventricular rate <100/min.

Drugs that restore and maintain sinus rhythm in AF:
1 Flecainide.
2 Sotalol.
3 Propafenone.

Ventricular tachycardia – key ECG features:
1 Ventricular rate >120/min.
2 Broad QRS complexes.

Ventricular tachycardia:
1 IHD.
2 MVP.
3 Dilated/hypertrophic cardiomyopathy.
4 Myocarditis.
5 Electrolyte disturbances.
6 Pro-arrhythmic drugs.

Accelerated idioventricular rhythm (slow form of VT):
1 Ventricular rate <120/min.
2 Broad QRS complexes.

Torsades de pointes (a variant of VT associated with a long QT interval):
1 Broad-complex tachycardia.
2 Variation in QRS axis ($\rightarrow$ the amplitude of QRS complexes undulates on the ECG strip).

Cardiac axis – key ECG features:
1 Normal axis = predominantly positive QRS complex in both leads I and II.
2 Left axis deviation = predominantly positive QRS complex in lead I and predominantly negative QRS complex in lead II.
3 Exclusion of left axis deviation = predominantly positive QRS complex in lead II excludes left axis deviation.

4 Right axis deviation = predominantly negative QRS complex in lead I and predominantly positive QRS complex in lead II.

5 Exclusion of right axis deviation = predominantly positive QRS complex in lead I excludes right axis deviation.

Left axis deviation – deviation of -30° to -90°; QRS negative in lead II:
1 LBBB.
2 Left anterior hemiblock.
3 Inferior wall infarction.
4 Left ventricular hypertrophy.
5 Horizontal heart.
6 Rhythm disturbances (WPW syndrome;[7] VT).
7 ASD (ostium primum type).

Right axis deviation – deviation of +90° to +180°; QRS negative in lead I:
1 RBBB.
2 Left posterior hemiblock.
3 Anterolateral wall infarction.
4 Right ventricular hypertrophy.
5 Vertical heart (in slender body build).
6 Rhythm disturbances (WPW syndrome).
7 ASD (ostium secundum type).
8 Dextrocardia.
9 Pulmonary disease.

Low voltage waves in all leads:
1 Obesity.
2 Constrictive pericarditis/pericardial effusion.
3 COPD (emphysema).
4 Hypothyroidism.

Inverted P waves:
1 Electrode misplacement.
2 Dextrocardia.
3 Retrograde atrial depolarisation (from atrial, junctional or ventricular ectopic foci):
   a Atrial ectopics.
   b AV junctional rhythm.
   c Ventricular ectopics (retrogradely conducted).
   d VT (retrogradely conducted).

---

7   In WPW syndrome, if the 'accessory' pathway lies on the right side of the heart, patient
     will have left axis deviation and vice versa.

Tall P waves (≥2.5 small squares) – also called 'P pulmonale':
1 Right atrial enlargement d/t any cause.

Wide (≥2 small squares across)/bifid P waves – also called 'P mitrale':
1 Left atrial enlargement d/t any cause.

Depolarisation from a focus near AV node – key ECG features:
1 P waves inverted in lead II.
2 Short PR interval.

Short PR interval (<0.12 sec/3 small squares):
1 AV junctional rhythm (AV junctional escape or premature beat/AV re-entry tachycardia).
2 Wolff–Parkinson–White's (WPW) syndrome.
3 Lown–Ganong–Levine's (LGL) syndrome.

Wolff–Parkinson–White's (WPW) syndrome – key ECG features:
1 Short PR interval.
2 Delta wave (slurred upstroke of the QRS complex).[8]

WPW syndrome – left-sided accessory pathway (bundle of Kent) – key ECG features:
1 Short PR interval.
2 Delta wave (slurred upstroke of the QRS complex).
3 Dominant R wave in leads V_1–V_3.
4 Right axis deviation.

WPW syndrome – right-sided accessory pathway – key ECG features:
1 Short PR interval.
2 Delta wave (slurred upstroke of the QRS complex).
3 Dominant S wave in leads V_1–V_3.
4 Left axis deviation.

WPW syndrome – arrhythmias caused:
1 SVT.
2 AF.
3 VF.

---

8   The region of the ventricle activated via the accessory pathway depolarises *slowly*. This gives rise to a slurred upstroke of the QRS complex called delta wave. Thereafter, rest of the ventricle is *rapidly* depolarised by the normally conducted wave of depolarisation via the AV node.

Lown–Ganong–Levine's syndrome (LGL) – key ECG features:
1 Short PR interval.
2 No delta wave.

Long PR interval (>0.2 sec/5 small squares):
1 Heart block:
   a 1st degree heart block.
   b 2nd degree heart block (Mobitz type 1 block – also called Wenckebach block).
2 IHD.
3 Acute rheumatic myocarditis.
4 Lyme disease.
5 Hypokalaemia.
6 Drugs (β-blockers; rate-limiting Ca^{2+} channel blockers; digoxin; quinidine).

Variable PR intervals:
2nd degree heart block:
   a PR interval gradually lengthens with each beat until one P wave fails to produce a QRS complex = Mobitz type-I block/also called Wenckebach block).
   b Fixed PR interval but occasionally a P wave fails to produce a QRS complex = Mobitz type-II block.
   c Alternate P waves are not followed by QRS complexes = 2:1 AV block.

3rd degree (complete) heart block:
   There is no relationship between P waves and QRS complexes + brady-cardia (ventricular foci usually discharge at a rate of 15–40/min) + broad QRS complexes.[9]

Young patient with 1st/2nd/3rd degree heart block:
1 Lyme disease – 2nd stage of illness (caused by the spirochaete *Borrelia burgdorferi*).[10]

Normal Q waves:
1 Small Q waves in the lateral leads – I, aVL, V_5 and V_6 – are normal and result from septal depolarisation from left to right.
2 A small Q wave with associated inverted T wave in lead III is also normal. Both may disappear on deep inspiration.

---

9 Any atrial rhythm can coexist with the 3rd degree heart block so that the P waves may be abnormal or even absent. A combination of bradycardia (15–40/min) and broad QRS complexes however should make one think about 3rd degree heart block.

10 Treatment is antibiotics. Some patients may also require temporary pacemaker.

Pathological Q waves – wide (>1 small square) or deep (>2 small squares/>25% of the height of the following R wave in depth):
1 MI.
2 Left ventricular hypertrophy.
3 Bundle branch block.
4 Pulmonary embolism ($S_IQ_{III}T_{III}$) – it rarely fulfils the width and depth criteria mentioned above.

Posterior MI – key ECG features:
1 R waves in leads V_1–V_3 (reciprocal of Q waves).
2 ST segment depression in leads V_1–V_3 (reciprocal of ST segment elevation).
3 Upright, tall T waves in leads V_1–V_3 (reciprocal of T wave inversion).

Height of R wave and depth of S wave – normal ECG findings:
1 The R wave increases in height from lead V_1 to V_6.
2 The R wave is smaller than the S wave in leads V_1 and V_2.
3 The R wave is bigger than the S wave in leads V_5 and V_6.
4 The tallest R wave does not exceed 25 mm in height.
5 The deepest S wave does not exceed 25 mm in depth.

Tall (>25 mm) R or deep (>25 mm) S waves in anterior chest leads:
1 Incorrect ECG calibration (should be 1 mV = 10 mm).
2 Ventricular hypertrophy (left/right).
3 Posterior wall MI.
4 Bundle branch block.
5 WPW syndrome.
6 Dextrocardia.

Left ventricular hypertrophy (LVH) – ECG criteria:
- R wave in V_5 or V_6 >25 mm.
- S wave in V_1 or V_2 >25 mm.
- Total of R wave in V_5 or V_6 + S wave in V_1 or V_2 >35 mm.

Left ventricular hypertrophy (LVH) with strain:
1 ST segment depression and T wave inversion in leads I, aVL and V_4–V_6 in addition to the above-mentioned criteria for LVH.

Right ventricular hypertrophy (RVH) – ECG criteria:
- Dominant R wave (bigger than the S wave) in V_1.
- Additional features present in some include:
  - Right bundle branch block.
  - Deep S wave in leads V_5 and V_6.
  - Right axis deviation.

Right ventricular hypertrophy (RVH) with strain:

1 ST segment depression and T wave inversion in leads V_1–V_3 in addition to the above-mentioned criteria for RVH.

Dominant R wave (bigger than the S wave) in V_1:

1 Right ventricular hypertrophy.
2 RBBB.
3 Posterior wall MI.
4 WPW syndrome (left-sided accessory pathway).[11]

Dextrocardia – key ECG features:

1 Progressive decrease in the R wave height across the anterior chest leads.[12]
2 Inverted P wave in lead I.
3 Right axis deviation.
4 ECG abnormalities will normalise when chest leads are applied to the 'right-sided' chest.

Small QRS complexes:

1 Physiological:
    a   Normal variant.
2 Mechanical:
    a   Incorrect ECG calibration (should be 1 mV = 10 mm).
3 Pathological (conditions that increase the distance between the heart and the chest electrodes):
    a   Obesity.
    b   Emphysema.
    c   Pericardial effusion.[13]

Wide QRS complexes (>0.12 sec/3 small squares):

1 Bundle branch block (right or left).
2 Ventricular rhythm.
3 Hyperkalaemia.

Left and right bundle branch blocks – key ECG features:
Mnemonic: **William Marrow**

---

11 Dominant R wave in V_1–V_3 indicates left-sided accessory pathway; dominant S wave in V_1–V_3 indicates right-sided accessory pathway.

12 Normally, there is a progressive increase in the R wave height across the anterior chest leads.

13 Pericardial effusion can also cause *electrical alternans* in which the heights of the R waves and/or T waves alternate from beat to beat. A combination of tachycardia, small QRS complexes and electrical alternans is a very specific, though insensitive, indicator of a pericardial tamponade.

- In LBBB, the QRS complex is broad and looks like a 'W' in lead V_1 and an 'M' in lead V_6 (**William**).
- In RBBB, the QRS complex is broad and looks like an 'M' in lead V_1 and a 'W' in lead V_6 (**Marrow**).

LBBB – the origin of 'W'[14] in lead V_1:
- Septal depolarisation occurs from right to left. This produces a small Q wave (the 1st downstroke) in lead V_1.
- Right ventricle depolarises normally producing an R wave (the central upstroke) in lead V_1.
- Left ventricle depolarises late from the right ventricle producing an S wave (the 2nd downstroke) in lead V_1.

LBBB – the origin of 'M' in lead V_6:
- Septal depolarisation occurs from right to left. This produces a small R wave (the 1st upstroke) in lead V_6.
- Right ventricle depolarises normally producing an S wave (the central downstroke) in lead V_6.
- Left ventricle depolarises late from the right ventricle producing an Ŕ wave (the 2nd upstroke) in lead V_6.

RBBB – the origin of 'M' in lead V_1:
- Septal depolarisation occurs from left to right. This produces a small R wave (the 1st upstroke) in lead V_1.
- Left ventricle depolarises normally producing an S wave (the central downstroke) in lead V_1.
- Right ventricle depolarises late from the left ventricle producing an Ŕ wave (the 2nd upstroke) in lead V_1.

RBBB – the origin of 'W' in lead V_6:
- Septal depolarisation occurs from right to left. This produces a small Q wave (the 1st downstroke) in lead V_6.
- Left ventricle depolarises normally producing an R wave (the central upstroke) in lead V_6.
- Right ventricle depolarises late from the left ventricle producing an S wave (the 2nd downstroke) in lead V_6.

Left bundle branch block (LBBB)[15] – almost always pathological:
1 IHD.

---

14 The first downstroke is a Q wave, the central upstroke is an R wave and the second downstroke is an S wave.

15 LBBB and RBBB do not require treatment *per se*. What is required is treatment of the underlying cause.

2 Left ventricular hypertrophy (d/t HTN; AS).
3 Cardiomyopathy.
4 Fibrosis of the conduction system.
5 Post valve replacement.
6 Right ventricular pacemaker.

VT with LBBB morphology:
1 Arrhythmogenic right ventricular cardiomyopathy (ARVC).
2 Right ventricular outflow tract VT.
3 Dilated cardiomyopathy.
4 Congenital cyanotic heart disease.

Right bundle branch block (RBBB) – may be a normal variant:
1 IHD.
2 Congenital/septal anomaly (Ebstein's anomaly; ASD).
3 Cardiomyopathy.
4 Pulmonary embolism (usually massive).

Incomplete[16] bundle branch block – key ECG features:
1 Left or right bundle branch morphology.
2 QRS complexes are not broad (<3 small squares wide).

Bifascicular block[17] – key ECG features:
1 RBBB + left axis deviation (d/t left anterior hemiblock).

Trifascicular block[18] – key ECG features:
1 RBBB + left axis deviation + 1st degree AV block (long PR interval).

Abnormally shaped QRS complexes (appear slurred or have an abnormal notch without being abnormally tall, small or wide):
1 Incomplete bundle branch block.
2 Fascicular block.
3 WPW syndrome.

ST segment elevation:
1 Acute MI (STEMI).
2 Left ventricular aneurysm (secondary to old MI).
3 Prinzmetal's (vasospastic) angina.

---

16 This develops when conduction down a bundle branch is *delayed* but not blocked.

17 RBBB + block of either fascicle (mostly left anterior hemiblock; left posterior hemiblock is extremely rare) = bifascicular block. If it is associated with syncopal attacks, permanent pacemaker is indicated; asymptomatic block generally doesn't require pacing.

18 Bifascicular block + 1st degree AV block = trifascicular block.

4 Pericarditis.
5 Aortic dissection (if it has involved the coronary arteries).
6 High take-off (normal variant).

ST segment depression:
1 IHD (NSTEMI; acute posterior wall MI; angina pectoris).
2 Ventricular hypertrophy with strain.
3 Antiarrhythmic drugs (e.g. digoxin; quinidine).

Acute MI – key ECG features:[19]
ST segment elevation + Q waves + T wave inversion.
OR
New onset LBBB.

STEMI – sequence of development of key ECG changes:
ST segment elevation accompanied, or even preceded, by tall hyperacute T waves are the earliest changes → over the next few hours or days, Q waves appear → T wave inversion.

Diagnosing acute MI:
At least two of the following three criteria should be met:
1 Suggestive history.
2 ECG changes.
3 ↑ cardiac enzyme levels.

Cardiac enzymes 'peak times' after acute MI:
1 Troponins peak after 12 hr.
2 CK peaks after 24 hr.
3 AST peaks after 30 hr.
4 LDH peaks after 48 hr.

↑ Cardiac troponins:
1 Cardiac pathology (MI; tachyarrhythmias; DC cardioversion; dilated/hypertrophic cardiomyopathy; myopericarditis).
2 Pulmonary pathology (pulmonary embolism; acute exacerbation of COPD).
3 CKD.
4 SAH.
5 Septicaemia.

---

19 ECG changes of acute MI may take a few hours to develop. A normal ECG, therefore, doesn't exclude acute MI.

Localisation of MI:
Leads containing ST segment elevation:
1 V_1–V_4 = anterior MI.
2 I, aVL, V_5–V_6 = lateral MI.
3 I, aVL, V_1–V_6 = anterolateral MI.
4 V_1–V_3 = anteroseptal MI.
5 II, III, aVF = inferior MI.
6 I, aVL, V_5–V_6, II, III, aVF = inferolateral MI.
7 V_1–V_3 showing dominant R wave, ST segment depression and tall upright T waves = acute posterior MI.
8 V_4R[20] = right ventricular MI.

Q wave vs. non-Q wave infarction:[21]
1 Whereas thrombolysis is the mainstay of treatment in cases of Q wave infarcts, the same has not been shown to improve prognosis in cases of non-Q wave infarcts. Glycoprotein IIb-IIIa inhibitors, however, are beneficial in selected cases of non-Q wave infarcts.
2 Non-Q wave infarcts appear to be at a higher risk of re-infarction. The 3-yr mortality, however, appears to be matchable.

Diagnosing left ventricular aneurysm (secondary to old MI):
1 Palpation: 'double impulse' in precordial palpation.
2 Auscultation: S_4.
3 CXR: a bulge on the cardiac outline.
4 Persistent ST segment elevation months after acute MI.
5 Echo confirmatory.

Prinzmetal's (vasospastic) angina – key ECG features:
1 ST segment elevation ± tall, hyperacute[22] T waves or T wave inversion only *during the episode* of chest pain. When chest pain normalises, ECG changes also revert back to normal.

Pericarditis – key ECG features:
1 'Saddle-shaped' (concave upward[23]) ST segment elevation in all leads except aVR and V_1, which show reciprocal ST segment depression.

---

20 To rule out right ventricular involvement in a case of acute MI, perform another ECG using right-sided chest leads. If ST segment elevation is shown in V_4R, it suggests right ventricular involvement.

21 Thinking that Q wave infarcts are always full thickness and non-Q wave infarcts are always subendocardial is something that has been disproved in postmortem studies. Therefore, terms like full thickness and subendocardial should better be avoided.

22 Ischaemic damage to the myocytes → K^+ release → localised hyperkalaemia → tall 'hyperacute' T waves.

23 In STEMI, ST segment is convex upward.

2 T wave inversion (unlike MI, it only develops when ST segment has already returned to the baseline).

3 No Q waves.

ST segment elevation (high take-off)[24] – key ECG features:
1 A high take-off ST segment always follows an S wave.
2 It is not associated with reciprocal ST segment depression.

Angina pectoris – key ECG features:
1 ST segment depression in the corresponding leads.
2 The depressed ST segment is 'horizontal' (as opposed to the down-sloping or 'reverse tick' ST segment seen with digoxin therapy).
3 T wave inversion.
4 No Q wave.

Abnormally tall T waves (generally, should be no more than half the size of the preceding QRS complex):
1 Normal variant.
2 Hyperkalaemia.
3 Acute MI.

Hyperkalaemia – key ECG features:
1 Tall 'tented' T waves. May also cause widening of the T waves so that the entire ST segment is incorporated into the upstroke of the T wave.
2 Flattening and even loss of the P wave.
3 Lengthening of the PR interval.
4 Widening of the QRS complex.
5 Arrhythmias.

Tall T waves in acute MI:
1 ST segment elevation accompanied, or even preceded by tall, hyperacute T waves (the earliest ECG changes of acute MI).
2 Acute posterior wall MI in leads V_1–V_3.

Abnormally small T waves:
1 Hypokalaemia.
2 Pericardial effusion.
3 Hypothyroidism.

Hypokalaemia – key ECG features:
1 Small T waves.
2 Prominent U waves.

---

24 High take-off ST segment is a normal variant and it represents 'early repolarisation'.

3 ST segment depression, 1st degree heart block (long PR interval) and peaked P waves may also be seen.

Abnormally prominent U waves:[25]

1 Hypokalaemia.

2 Hypercalcaemia (short QT interval ± prominent U waves)

3 Hyperthyroidism (sinus tachycardia ± prominent U waves)

Hypothyroidism – key ECG features:

1 Sinus bradycardia (the most characteristic finding) + small QRS complexes and T waves.

T wave inversion:

Physiological in:

1 Leads aVR and V1.

2 Lead V1–V2 (in young persons).

3 Lead V1–V3 (in blacks).

4 Lead III.[26]

Pathological (if found in leads other than the above):

Common causes:

1 IHD (MI; angina pectoris[27]).

2 Ventricular hypertrophy with strain.

3 Digoxin toxicity.

Uncommon causes:

1 Arrhythmias (repolarisation abnormalities following a paroxysmal tachycardia; bundle branch block).

2 Permanent ventricular pacing.

3 Mitral valve prolapse.

4 Pericarditis.

5 Pulmonary embolism.

6 Hyperventilation.

7 Subarachnoid haemorrhage.

---

25 Presence of U waves is normal. They probably represent interventricular septal repolarisation. They are most clearly seen in leads V_2–V_4.

26 Both T wave inversion and a small Q wave can be seen normally; both of these can disappear if ECG is repeated with patient's breath held in inspiration.

27 T wave inversion *during* an ischaemic episode may get normalised (upright) transiently. This is called T wave pseudonormalisation.

Short (<0.35 sec) QT interval:[28,29]

1 Hypercalcaemia.
2 Hyperthermia.
3 Digoxin effect.

Prolonged (>0.43 sec) QT interval:
Common causes:

1 Commonest cause (90%): hereditary syndromes (*autosomal dominant* – Romano–Ward's syndrome; *autosomal recessive* – Jervell and Lange-Nielsen's syndrome).
2 Hypocalcaemia.
3 Hypothermia.
4 Drugs [antiarrhythmic drugs (e.g. procainamide; flecainide; quinidine); TCAs].[30]
5 Acute myocarditis.

Less common causes:

1 Acute MI.
2 Hypertrophic cardiomyopathy.
3 Cerebral injury.

Inverted U waves:

1 U waves follow T waves. U waves are therefore inverted in conditions that cause T wave inversion.

Pacing and the ECG:

1 Atrial pacing (via an atrial lead):
  a The pacing spike (generated by the pacemaker) will be followed by a P wave and a normal (narrow) QRS complex.
2 Ventricular pacing (via a ventricular lead):
  a The pacing spike will be followed by a broad QRS complex (because the depolarisation is not carried by the normal, fast-conduction pathways).
3 Dual-chamber sequential pacing (there are two leads – one atrial and the other ventricular):

---

28 QT interval should not include the U wave. Since U wave can easily be mistaken for a T wave, QT interval should always be measured in aVL, where the U waves are normally least prominent.

29 The duration of QT interval varies according to the patient's heart rate – the faster the heart rate, the shorter the QT interval. Thus in cases of tachycardia, the duration of QT interval should be corrected as per this formula: $QT_c = QT/\sqrt{RR}$ where QT_c is the *corrected* QT interval, QT is the *measured* QT interval and RR is the *measured* RR interval (all in seconds).

30 Drug-induced QT-interval prolongation → torsades de pointes → ventricular fibrillation → sudden cardiac death.

a P wave will be followed by a pacing spike from the ventricular lead and a broad QRS complex.

Indications of biventricular pacing:
1 Clinical (severe NYHA class III–IV failure despite optimal drug therapy).
2 ECG (QRS >130 msec).
3 Echo (LV end-diastolic diameter >55 mm; LV ejection fraction <35%).

ECG artefacts:
1 External electrical interference (e.g. from other electrical appliances, especially home appliances).
2 Patient movement ($\rightarrow$ skeletal muscle activity is also picked up on the ECG).
3 Electrode misplacement.
4 Incorrect calibration.[31]
5 Incorrect paper speed.[32]

Indications of permanent pacing:
1 3rd degree block:
  a Symptomatic 3rd degree block (associated with an episode of syncope or presyncope).
  b Asymptomatic 3rd degree block if ventricular rate is <40/min or pauses >3 sec.
2 2nd degree block (if it is associated with an episode of symptomatic bradycardia).[33]
3 Bifascicular or trifascicular block (if it is associated with an episode of syncope or documented intermittent failure of the remaining fascicle).
4 Symptomatic bradycardia:
  a Sick-sinus syndrome (if it has caused symptomatic bradycardia).
  b Carotid sinus syndrome (if it has caused symptomatic bradycardia).
  c Vasovagal syndrome (if it has caused symptomatic bradycardia).

---

31 Normal calibration: 1 mV = 1 cm, i.e. a voltage of 1 mV makes the recording needle move 1 cm. If ECG shows too big or too small waves, the first thing to check is the size of the calibration mark. The problem simply could be an incorrect calibration. If calibration mark is correct and yet the QRS complexes are so big that they will not fit the ECG paper, change the calibration to adjust their amplitude.

32 Normal: 25 mm/s (one small square = 0.04 sec). At 50 mm/s speed, the waves will double in width.

33 Patients with 2nd and 3rd degree AV blocks who do not have a permanent pacemaker should be considered for a temporary pacemaker if they are to undergo a surgical procedure under general anaesthesia.

Indications of automatic implantable cardioverter defibrillators (AICDs) – NICE guidelines:
1 Primary prevention:
  a Post MI with:
    i   Non-sustained VT on 24-hr tape.
    ii Inducible VT on electrophysiological studies (EPS).
    iii Left ventricular EF <35%.
  b Familial cardiac conditions:
    i   Long QT interval.
    ii Brugada's syndrome (RBBB + down-sloping ST elevation in V_1).
    iii Hypertrophic cardiomyopathy.
    iv Arrhythmogenic right ventricular dysplasia.
    v Following repair of Fallot's tetralogy.
2 Secondary prevention:
  a VT or VF → cardiac arrest.
  b VT → significant haemodynamic compromise.
  c Sustained VT with EF <35%.

Indications for coronary angiography in cases of NSTEMI:
1 ↑ serum troponin T or I.
2 NSTEMI + malignant ventricular arrhythmias.
3 NSTEMI + LVF.

Bad clinical signs during an arrhythmia:
1 IHD.
2 LVF/CCF.
3 Excessive tachycardia (>200/min for narrow-complex tachycardia and >150/min for broad-complex tachycardia).
4 Excessive bradycardia (<40/min).
5 Low systolic BP (<90 mmHg).
6 Low cardiac output (as indicated by poor peripheral perfusion and impaired conscious level.

ECG predictors of asystole:
1 Recent asystole.
2 2nd degree AV block (Mobitz type II).
3 3rd degree AV block with broad QRS complexes.
4 Ventricular pauses >3.0 sec.

4 Pulmonology

Appearance suggestive of blood gas disturbance:
1 Hypoxic: blue hands and tongue, i.e. central cyanosis, restless, confused, drowsy or unconscious.
2 CO_2 retention: warm hands, bounding pulse, dilated veins on hands and face, twitching of facial muscles, drowsy.
3 Hypocapnia: hyperventilation, paraesthesia around lips, dizzy.

Low respiratory rate (<10/min):
1 ↑ ICP.
2 CO_2 narcosis (i.e. severe hypercapnia).
3 Drugs (opiates; benzodiazepines; alcohol).

Sputum:
1 Serous (clear and frothy):
  a Acute pulmonary oedema.
2 Mucoid (white):
  a Chronic bronchitis.
3 Purulent (yellow or green):
  a Pneumonia.
  b TB.
  c Bronchiectasis.
  d Lung abscess.
4 Mucopurulent:
  a Chronic bronchitis with secondary infection.
5 Thick tenacious sputum (difficult to cough up):
  a Bronchial asthma.
6 Foul-smelling sputum (suggests anaerobic infection):
  a Lung abscess.
  b Bronchiectasis.

Frank haemoptysis (pure blood is coughed up):
1 TB.
2 Bronchiectasis.
3 Pulmonary infarction.
4 MS.

Blood-stained sputum (blood is mixed with sputum):
1 TB.
2 Ca. lung.

Blood-streaked sputum (blood is present on the side of the sputum):
1 Chronic bronchitis.

Rusty sputum (golden-yellow-coloured sputum d/t degradation of Hb):
1 Pneumococcal pneumonia.

Musculoskeletal chest pain:
1 Rib cage problem (costochondritis; rib fracture; rib metastases).
2 Nerve problem (spinal root compression; herpes zoster).

Expiratory polyphonic, high-pitched wheeze – loud rhonchus audible without a stethoscope (suggests small airway narrowing):
1 Bronchial asthma.
2 Asthmatic bronchitis.
3 Anaphylaxis.
4 LVF and pulmonary oedema (cardiac asthma).

Inspiratory monophonic wheeze (suggests large airway obstruction):
Tracheal obstruction 'lesion above carina' may be life threatening as neither lung can be ventilated.
1 Laryngeal obstruction (*see* 'stridor').
2 Tracheal obstruction:
  a Blunt trauma to trachea.
  b Tracheal stenosis after ventilation.
  c Tracheal tumour.
  d Exogenous compression on trachea (by mediastinal mass; oesophageal mass).

Expiratory monophonic wheeze (suggests large airway obstruction):
1 Same as 'inspiratory monophonic wheeze'.

Stridor (suggests obstruction in or near larynx):
Unlike rhonchus, which is louder during expiration, stridor is louder during inspiration; also the intensity of stridor decreases as one auscultates away from the centre:
1 Inflammation/infection d/t epiglottitis, croup, anaphylaxis, etc (→ laryngeal oedema).
2 Inhaled foreign body.
3 Tumour (laryngeal papilloma).
4 Rapidly progressive laryngomalacia.

Epistaxis:
1 Local nasal pathology (the usual cause).
2 Hypertension.

3 Bleeding/clotting disorder.

Physiologic types of respiration:
1 Abdominothoracic respiration: physiological in males and babies.
2 Thoracoabdominal respiration: physiological in females.

Abnormal breathing:
1 Pure thoracic breathing:
  a Peritonitis.
  b ↑ intra-abdominal pressure.
2 Pure abdominal breathing:
  a Pleuritis.
  b Intercostal paralysis.
  c Ankylosing spondylitis.
3 Acidotic breathing:
  a Metabolic acidosis (ARF; DKA; lactic acidosis; salicylic acid poisoning).
4 Cheyne–Stokes' breathing (↓ sensitivity of the respiratory centre to CO_2):
  a Heart pathology (LVF).
  b Brain pathology (↑ ICP; brainstem lesion).
  c Drugs (narcotic overdose).

Chest deformities – barrel-shaped chest (↑ AP diameter):
1 Emphysema (↑ risk if disease starts before the age of 30).
2 Kyphosis.

Chest deformities – pectus carinatum
(pigeon chest – prominence of sternum, often associated with indrawing of ribs causing Harrison's sulci above the costal margins):
1 Developmental anomaly.
2 Complication of any chronic respiratory disease like emphysema.
3 Rickets.

Chest deformities – pectus excavatum
(funnel chest – localised depression of the lower end of the sternum):
1 Developmental anomaly.

Chest deformities – Harrison's sulcus
(horizontal groove d/t indrawing of the ribs where diaphragm is attached):
1 Complication of any chronic respiratory disease like emphysema.

Chest deformities – kyphosis:
1 Congenital.
2 Anterior collapse of spinal vertebrae (d/t spinal TB, etc).

Chest deformities – scoliosis:
1 Congenital.
2 TB.
3 Neuromuscular disease.
4 Previous surgery.

Chest deformities – local bulging of the chest wall:
1 Rib problem (fracture/malunion of the ribs).
2 Pleural problem (pleural effusion; pneumothorax).

Chest deformities – local flattening or retraction of the chest wall:
1 Fibrosis/collapse of lung.
2 Pneumonectomy.

Chest deformities – absence of part of bony chest cage:
1 Congenital (Poland's syndrome).
2 Post surgery.

Pulsations in the interscapular region (seen when the patient bends forward):
1 Coarctation of aorta.

Unilaterally reduced chest movements:
1 Pleural pathology (pleural effusion; pneumothorax).
2 Lung pathology (consolidation; collapse; fibrosis).
3 Chest cage pathology (fractured ribs; flail segment; previous thoracoplasty).

Bilaterally reduced chest expansion (normal is >5 cm; <2 cm is abnormal):
1 Obesity.
2 Lung pathology (emphysema; bronchial asthma; diffuse pulmonary fibrosis).
3 Chest cage pathology (ankylosing spondylitis).
4 Neuromuscular pathology (GB syndrome; multiple sclerosis; MND; muscular dystrophy and other rarer myopathies).

Mediastinal pull towards the diseased side – both trachea and apex beat are shifted:
1 Lung pathology (collapse; fibrosis).

Mediastinal push away from the diseased side – both trachea and apex beat are shifted:
1 Pleural pathology (pleural effusion; pneumothorax).

Pneumothorax ordinarily *pulls* the mediastinum; tension pneumothorax, however, *pushes* the mediastinum.

Tracheal shift alone may be d/t thyroid pathology.

Signs of consolidation:
1 Chest movements decreased.
2 Trachea is central.
3 Percussion note is impaired.
4 Breath sounds are bronchial in character.
5 Coarse crepitations may be audible.
6 VF ↑; VR ↑; whispering pectoriloquy positive.

↑ Vocal fremitus:
(Mnemonic – CCC)
1 **C**onsolidation.
2 **C**avitation.
3 **C**ollapse with patent main bronchus.

↓ Vocal fremitus:
1 Pleural pathology (pleural effusion; pneumothorax).
2 Collapse with obstructed main bronchus.

Percussion notes:
1 Resonant:
  a Produced by percussing over normal lung tissue.
2 Hyper-resonant:
  a Pneumothorax.
  b Emphysema (over a large bulla).
3 Tympanitic:
  a Produced by percussing over hollow viscus, e.g. empty stomach.
4 Impaired note:
  a Normally present over the lung–heart and lung–liver borders.
  b Lung fibrosis.
5 Dull note:
  a Normally present over solid organs, e.g. liver and heart.
  b Lung pathology (consolidation; collapse – some cases; pulmonary oedema).
  c Pleural pathology (plural thickening, e.g. d/t mesothelioma).
6 Stony-dull note:
  a Pleural effusion.

Diminished breath sounds:
1 Poor respiratory effort.

2 Pleural pathology (pleural effusion; pneumothorax; pleural thickening, e.g. d/t mesothelioma).
3 Collapse with obstructed main bronchus.
4 Emphysema (generalised diminished breath sounds).
5 Severe asthma (d/t severe bronchoconstriction).
6 Elevated hemidiaphragm (say d/t phrenic nerve palsy).

Bronchial breathing:
1 Normally heard over the trachea and the upper part of midline.
2 CCC: consolidation; cavitation; collapse with patent main bronchus.

Amphoric type of bronchial breathing (sound produced by blowing across the top of a bottle):
1 Tension pneumothorax (some cases).

Vesicular breathing with prolonged expiration:
1 Bronchial asthma.
2 COPD.

Rhonchi:
1 Bronchial asthma.
2 COPD.

Forced expiratory time (normal <4 sec):
1 Bronchial asthma.
2 COPD.

Fixed rhonchus (constant low-pitched rhonchus):
1 Obstruction of a major bronchus, e.g. d/t foreign body or tumour.

Pan-inspiratory crepitations (heard d/t the bubbling of air through secretions in the bronchi and alveoli):
1 Chronic bronchitis.
2 Bronchiectasis.
3 Resolving pneumonia.
4 Tuberculous cavity.
5 Lung abscess.
6 Emphysema.

End-inspiratory crepitations (heard d/t explosive reopening of thickened alveoli):
1 Pulmonary oedema.
2 Fibrosing alveolitis.

Unlike pleural rub, crepitations are always inspiratory and they may change their character on coughing. Pleural rub is heard at the end of inspiration and the beginning of expiration; it never changes its character on coughing; characteristically, its intensity increases on pressing the stethoscope.

Coarse crepitations (bubbly crackles):
1 Bronchiectasis.

Positive coin test:
1 Tension pneumothorax.

Succussion splash:
1 Hydro-pneumothorax.

Don't confuse it with gastric succussion splash.

Acute dyspnoea – onset over seconds:
1 Anaphylaxis.
2 Pulmonary embolism.
3 Pneumothorax.
4 Foreign body inhalation.

Acute dyspnoea + wheeze ± cough:
1 Anaphylaxis.
2 Asthma.
3 COPD.
4 Acute viral or bacterial bronchitis.
5 Acute LVF.

Cough + pink frothy sputum:
1 Acute pulmonary oedema.
2 MS.

Frank haemoptysis/sputum streaking:
1 Infection (pulmonary TB; acute viral or bacterial bronchitis; bronchiectasis; lung abscess).
2 Ca. lung.
3 Pulmonary infarction.
4 URT abnormalities (nasal polyps; laryngeal ca.; pharyngeal tumours).
5 AVM.
6 Autoimmune diseases (Wegener's granulomatosis; Goodpasture's syndrome).

Hoarseness:
1 Vocal cord pathology:
   a Vocal cord paresis (d/t recurrent laryngeal nerve/vagal nerve trauma; malignancy – thyroid; pharynx; oesophagus; bronchus; TB; MS; syringomyelia; polio; idiopathic in 15% cases).
   b Nodules on cord (singer's nodes)/granulomata on cord (d/t TB; sarcoid; Wegener's; syphilis).
2 Laryngeal pathology (voice abuse; laryngitis; ca. larynx).
3 Nerve pathology (recurrent laryngeal nerve palsy/10th nerve palsy).
4 Endocrine pathology (myxoedema; acromegaly).
5 Autoimmune pathology (sicca syndrome).
6 Functional (at times of stress; able to cough normally).

'Exudative' pleural effusion (protein >3 g/dL):
1 Infective (parapneumonic [sterile]; empyema; TB; viral, etc).
2 Pulmonary infarction.
3 Connective tissue disorders (SLE; RA).
4 Malignancy (ca. lung; metastases; lymphoma; leukaemia; mesothelioma).

Light's criteria for exudative pleural effusion:
1 Protein:
   a Pleural fluid protein to serum protein ratio >0.5.
2 LDH:
   a Pleural fluid LDH to serum LDH ratio >0.6.
   b Pleural fluid LDH $>^2/_3$ the normal upper limit of serum LDH.

Low pH and low glucose pleural effusion:
1 Infective (parapneumonic/empyema/tuberculous).
2 Connective tissue disorders (SLE; RA).
3 Malignancy.
4 Oesophageal rupture ($\downarrow$ pH; $\downarrow$ glucose; $\uparrow$ amylase).

'Transudative' pleural effusion (protein <3 g/dL):
1 CCF.
2 Hypoproteinaemia (d/t any reason).
3 Meigs' syndrome (can be exudative).
4 Uncommon causes (myxoedema; primary pulmonary hypertension; pericarditis; SVC obstruction; peritoneal dialysis).

'Haemorrhagic' pleural effusion:
1 Malignancy (ca. lung; metastases; lymphoma; leukaemia; mesothelioma).
2 TB.
3 Pulmonary infarction.

Indications for tube thoracostomy:
1 Frank pus.
2 Organisms seen on staining or C/S of the pleural fluid.
3 Recurrence after two therapeutic aspirations.
4 Loculated fluid (decortication may be required).

Pneumothorax:
1 Spontaneous:
  a Primary (no lung pathology): usually occurs in smokers d/t rupture of the apical pleural plebs; recurs in 50% cases.
  b Secondary (to some lung pathology): COPD; TB.
2 Traumatic:
  a RTA.
  b Iatrogenic (pleural/transthoracic aspiration; insertion of CVP line/ double-lumen catheter).
3 Tension pneumothorax:
  a Iatrogenic (resuscitation; mechanical ventilation).

Dry cough:
1 Pharyngeal disease (pharyngitis).
2 Laryngeal disease (laryngitis; laryngeal paralysis).
3 Alveolar disease (fibrosing alveolitis).
4 GORD.
5 Drugs (ACEI therapy).

Productive cough:
1 Infections (tracheitis; acute/chronic bronchitis; bronchiectasis; pneumonia; TB; lung abscess).
2 Malignancy.
3 Postnasal drip.
4 Asthma.
5 Pulmonary oedema (d/t cardiac or non-cardiac causes).

Acute cough (<3 weeks):
1 URTI.
2 Pneumonia.
3 Pulmonary embolism.
4 Heart failure ($\rightarrow$ pulmonary oedema).

Chronic cough (>3 weeks):
1 Postnasal drip.
2 GORD.
3 Chronic bronchitis.
4 Bronchial asthma.

5 Bronchial carcinoma.

Haemoptysis:
1 Infections (TB; pneumonia; chronic bronchitis; bronchiectasis; lung abscess).
2 Malignancy/adenoma.
3 Pulmonary infarction.
4 MS.
5 Goodpasture's syndrome.
6 AVM.
7 Bleeding disorder.

Bronchiectasis:
1 Infection:
   a Viral (measles; whooping cough; influenza).
   b Bacterial (TB; *S. aureus*; Klebsiella).
   c Fungal (ABPA).
2 Congenital disorders (cystic fibrosis; Kartagener's syndrome/primary ciliary dyskinesia).
3 Foreign body.

Pulmonary nodules:
1 Tumour (ca. lung; metastases; adenoma).
2 Bacterial infection (lung abscess).
3 Fungal infection (aspergilloma).
4 Worm infestation (hydatid cyst).
5 Rarely (AVM; hamartoma).

Type-I respiratory failure:[1]
1 Bronchial asthma.
2 Pneumonia.
3 Pulmonary embolism.
4 Pulmonary oedema.
5 Alveolitis (allergic/fibrosing).

Type-II respiratory failure:
1 COPD (chronic bronchitis; emphysema; late stage of acute severe attack of bronchial asthma).
2 Depression of the respiratory centre (usually the result of sedative drugs overdosage).
3 Chest cage problem (severe kyphoscoliosis).

---

1 Respiratory failure: PaO_2 <8 kPa (60 mmHg) or $PaCO_2$ >6.5 kPa (50 mmHg). Type-I: PaO_2 ↓; $PaCO_2$ N or ↓; Type-II: PaO_2 ↓; $PaCO_2$ ↑.

4 Muscle problem (respiratory muscles paralysis).

Features of hypercapnia:
1 Symptoms: headache; sweating; muscle twitching; drowsiness.
2 Signs: warm extremities with engorged veins and bounding pulse; flapping tremors; papilloedema; engorged retinal veins.

Complications of COPD:
1 Pulmonary bullae ($\rightarrow$ spontaneous pneumothorax).
2 Type-II respiratory failure ($\rightarrow$ secondary polycythaemia).
3 Pulmonary hypertension ($\rightarrow$ cor pulmonale $\rightarrow$ right heart failure).

Interstitial lung disease:
1 Environmental (asbestosis; pneumoconiosis; extrinsic allergic alveolitis).
2 Interstitial pneumonitis/hypersensitivity pneumonitis.
3 Iatrogenic (drugs like amiodarone, antibiotics, etc; radiotherapy).
4 Connective tissue disorders.
5 Sarcoidosis.
6 Systemic sclerosis.

Drug-induced pulmonary fibrosis:
1 CVS drugs: amiodarone.
2 Antibiotics: ethambutol; minocycline; nitrofurantoin.
3 DMARDs: methotrexate; penicillamine; azathioprine.
4 Immunosuppressive agents: bleomycin; busulfan cyclophosphamide; chlorambucil.
5 Methysergide.

Young patient with a mixed obstructive and restrictive defect on PFTs:
1 Most probably histiocytosis X.

Pulmonary eosinophilia/eosinophilic pneumonia:
1 Infective:
    a Worms (*Ascaris lumbricoides*; *Ankylostoma duodenale*; *Strongyloides stercoralis*).
    b Parasite (filaria).
    c Fungus (ABPA in an asthmatic).
2 Non-infective:
    a Hypereosinophilic syndrome (none of the above + eosinophil count $>1.5 \times 10^9$/L + eosinophil infiltration of lungs, heart, liver, bones and nervous system).
    b Smoke inhalation.
3 Idiopathic (Löffler's syndrome).
4 Drugs (nitrofurantoin; sulfasalazine; imipramine).

Pulmonary vasculitis:
1 Recurrent pulmonary embolism.
2 Ulcerative colitis.
3 Behçet's syndrome.
4 Churg–Strauss' syndrome.
5 Giant cell arteritis.
6 Takayasu's arteritis.

Complications of ca. lung:[2]
Nerves involved:
1 Phrenic nerve ($\to$ raised hemidiaphragm).
2 Recurrent laryngeal nerve ($\to$ hoarseness of voice).
3 Pancoast's tumour $\to$ sympathetic trunk ($\to$ Horner's syndrome); C8, T1 and T2; 1st and 2nd ribs.

'Pipes' involved:
1 Trachea ($\to$ SOB; stridor).
2 Oesophagus ($\to$ dysphagia).
3 SVC ($\to$ chest varicosities).

Paraneoplastic:
1 Endocrine (PTH; ACTH; ADH).
2 Neurological (Eaton–Lambert's syndrome; polymyositis).
3 Haematological (thrombosis; phlebitis).

CXR – homogeneous well-defined lung opacity:
1 Lung pathology (consolidation d/t lobar pneumonia; collapsed lobe/lung; pulmonary infarction; dense pulmonary fibrosis).
2 Pneumonectomy.
3 Pleural pathology (pleural effusion; empyema).

CXR – diffuse poorly defined hazy opacity:
1 Pulmonary oedema (cardiogenic; fluid overload; ARDS).
2 Pulmonary haemorrhage.
3 Infection (viral pneumonia; gram-negative pneumonia).
4 Alveolar cell carcinoma.

CXR – round opacity/opacities >5 mm in diameter:
1 Neoplasia (benign tumour; ca. lung; metastases).

---

2 Can present as pneumonia, collapse or pleural effusion, with clubbing. Metastases to liver, brain and lymph nodes.

2 Infection ('rounded' pneumonia;[3] lung abscess; TB granuloma; hydatid cyst; histoplasmosis).

3 Rheumatoid nodule.

4 Wegener's granuloma.

5 AVM.

CXR – multiple nodular (2–5 mm) shadows and miliary mottling (<2 mm):
1 Granulomatous diseases (miliary tuberculosis; sarcoidosis).
2 Interstitial lung disease (pneumoconiosis).
3 Past infection (chicken-pox).
4 Metastases.
5 Mitral stenosis with pulmonary hypertension.
6 Histiocytosis X (eosinophilic granuloma).

CXR – increased linear markings:[4]
1 Interstitial fibrosis.
2 Interstitial (i.e. pulmonary) oedema.
3 Bronchiectasis.
4 Lymphangitis carcinomatosis.

CXR – upper-lobe pulmonary fibrosis:
1 Granulomatous disease (TB; sarcoidosis; histiocytosis X).
2 Occupational disease (pneumoconiosis; silicosis).
3 Extrinsic allergic alveolitis.
4 Fungal infection (ABPA).
5 Ankylosing spondylitis.

CXR – lower-lobe pulmonary fibrosis:
1 Bronchiectasis.
2 Cryptogenic fibrosing alveolitis (CFA).
3 Asbestosis.
4 Iatrogenic (drugs; radiation).
5 CT disorder (RA; systemic sclerosis).
6 Sarcoidosis.

CXR – cavitation:
1 Bullae.
2 Infection (pneumonias [*S. aureus*; *Klebsiella pneumoniae*; pseudomonas; anaerobes]; abscess; TB; histoplasmosis; hydatid disease).
3 Malignancy (benign; squamous cell ca.; metastases).

---

3   E.g. Klebsiella pneumonia, which produces multiple cavitating opacities especially in the upper lobes in an elderly person.

4   Indicates thickening of the interstitial tissue.

4 Fibrosis (progressive massive fibrosis [PMF]; honeycomb lung [systemic sclerosis]; sarcoidosis).
5 Nodules (pneumoconiosis; RA).
6 Vascular pathology (pulmonary embolism; vasculitides [Wegener's granulomatosis; Churg–Strauss' syndrome]).

CXR – bilaterally symmetrical dark lungs:
1 COPD.
2 Asthma.

CXR – single dark lung:
1 Pneumothorax.
2 Bulla.[5]
3 Mastectomy.

CXR – abnormal hilar shadowing:
1 Granulomatous disease (primary TB; sarcoidosis).
2 Malignancy (ca. lung; metastases; Hodgkin's or non-Hodgkin's lymphoma).
3 Prominent pulmonary artery (d/t pulmonary embolus/hypertension).

CXR – calcified lymph nodes:
1 TB.
2 Silicosis.
3 Carcinoid syndrome.

CXR – calcified pleura:
1 TB.
2 Haemothorax; recurrent pneumothorax; empyema.
3 Asbestosis.

CXR – calcified lung parenchyma:
1 Granulomatous diseases (TB; sarcoidosis).
2 Occupational diseases (pneumoconiosis; Caplan's syndrome; asbestosis; silicosis).
3 Infection (healed chicken pox pneumonia in adulthood; hydatid disease; schistosomiasis; coccidioidomycosis; histoplasmosis).
4 Malignancy (pulmonary metastases).

CXR – upper mediastinal widening:
1 Retrosternal goitre.

---

5 Loss of lung markings inside a lucent, thin-rimmed circular region (usually in a known case of COPD).

2 Thymoma.
3 Neoplasia (teratoma – benign or malignant; lymphadenopathy d/t ca. lung, metastases, Hodgkin's or non-Hodgkin's lymphoma).
4 Kinked aorta/aortic aneurysm.

CXR – fleeting lung shadows:
1 Wegener's granulomatosis.

↑ O_2 affinity – shift of O_2 dissociation curve to the right:
1 ↑ temperature.
2 Metabolic acidosis (↓ pH; ↑ H^+).
3 Respiratory acidosis (↓ pH; ↑ $PaCO_2$).
4 ↑ 2,3-DPG (secondary to high altitude, chronic anaemia).

↓ Gas transfer factor (TL_{CO}[6] and K_{CO}[7]):
1 COPD.
2 Restrictive airway disease (interstitial lung disease).
3 Pneumonia.
4 Pulmonary oedema.
5 Pulmonary embolism.
6 Pulmonary hypertension.
7 Pneumonectomy.
8 Anaemia.
9 AVM.
10 Lymphangitis carcinomatosa.

↑ Gas transfer factor (TL_{CO} and K_{CO}):
1 Exercise.
2 Asthma (when asymptomatic).
3 Pulmonary haemorrhage.
4 Polycythaemia.
5 Left-to-right shunt (e.g. ASD) with consequent increased pulmonary blood flow.
6 Thoracic cage deformities (may be normal).

---

6   TL_{CO}: total lung carbon monoxide transfer factor.
7   K_{CO}: corrected carbon monoxide transfer factor.

Lung function tests:

Spirometry	Obstructive airway disease[1]	Restrictive airway disease
FEV$_1$ (forced expiratory volume in one second)	↓↓	↓
FVC (forced vital capacity)	↓	↓↓
FEV$_1$/FVC	<70% (normal 70–80%)	>80%
TLC (total lung capacity)	↑ (d/t gas trapping)	↓
RV (residual volume)	↑	↓
TL$_{CO}$ (total lung CO transfer factor)	↓	↓
K$_{CO}$ (corrected CO transfer factor)	↓	↓[2]

1 Obstructive airway disease includes: COPD (chronic bronchitis; emphysema); asthma; bronchiectasis.
2 Exceptions include pulmonary haemorrhage (↑); neuromuscular defects/thoracic cage defects/pneumonectomy (unchanged or ↑).

Asthma – lung function tests:
1 ↓ FEV$_1$.
2 ↓ FEV$_1$/FVC ratio.
3 Salbutamol therapy → ↑ PEFR and FEV$_1$ (>25% variation in PEFR).
4 ↑ lung volume (↑ TLC; ↑ RV).
5 Unlike COPD, ↑ TL$_{CO}$ and ↑ K$_{CO}$.

5 Gastroenterology and hepatology

Red pharynx and tonsils:
1 Viral infection (viral tonsillitis; infectious mononucleosis – also called glandular fever – caused by Epstein–Barr virus).
2 Bacterial infection (acute follicular tonsillitis complicated by quinsy, retropharyngeal abscess or scarlet fever; meningococcal meningitis).
3 Agranulocytosis (e.g. caused by carbimazole).

Oral lesions:
1 Traumatic ulceration.
2 Aphthous ulcers (with associated lymph node enlargement).
3 Infection (vesicles in herpes simplex; creamy white plaques in candidiasis).
4 Atrophic or fissured tongue d/t vitamin deficiency (B_{12}/riboflavin/nicotinic acid).
5 Carious teeth.
6 Hereditary haemorrhagic telangiectasia (Osler–Weber–Rendu's syndrome).
7 Peri-oral pigmentation (not the tongue) – Peutz–Jeghers' syndrome (associated with intestinal polyps).

Pigmentation of the mucous membrane of the oral cavity:
1 Isolated finding.
2 Peutz–Jeghers' syndrome (associated with familial polyposis of small intestine).
3 Addison's disease.
4 Haemochromatosis.

White oral plaques:
1 Candidiasis.
2 Leucoplakia.
3 Hairy leucoplakia.
4 Condylomata latum of secondary syphilis.
5 Squamous cell carcinoma.

Recurrent belching:
1 Anxiety.

Superadded herpes labialis:
1 Malaria.
2 Pneumococcal pneumonia.

Angular stomatitis:
1 Iron/riboflavin deficiency.
2 Ill-fitting dentures.

Hypertrophied gums:
1 Phenytoin therapy.
2 Pregnancy.
3 AML.

Bleeding gums:
1 Leukaemias.
2 Thrombocytopenia.
3 Scurvy.

Yellow–grey staining of teeth:
1 Tetracycline therapy in early childhood.

Black hairy tongue:
1 Fungal infection.

Raw beef tongue:
1 Vitamin B_{12} deficiency.

Magenta tongue:
1 Riboflavin deficiency.

Enlarged tongue:
1 Amyloidosis.
2 Acromegaly.
3 Thyroid pathology (myxoedema; cretinism).

Bald tongue (atrophy of the papillae):
1 Nutritional deficiency (iron; riboflavin; niacin; pyridoxine; B_{12}).

Glossitis:
1 Nutritional deficiency (iron; riboflavin; niacin; pyridoxine; B_{12}).
2 Infection (syphilis).
3 Corrosives/inhalational burns.

Tonsils:
Yellow follicular exudate:
1 Streptococcal tonsillitis.

**White–green membrane covering the tonsils – membrane removal →
bleeding:**
  1 Diphtheria.

Scaphoid (sunken) abdomen:
  1 Starvation.
  2 Wasting disease (like malignancy).

Generalised abdominal distension:
  1 Fat (obesity).
  2 Fluid (ascites).
  3 Faeces (intestinal obstruction).
  4 Flatus.
  5 Foetus (pregnancy); fibroids; large ovarian cyst.

Umbilicus is sunken only in obesity. In other conditions, it is either flat or
everted.

In ascites, umbilicus is slit-like transversely, and at its normal position, in
contrast to ovarian cyst in which umbilicus is slit-like vertically, and displaced
upwards.

Poor intestinal movements:
  1 Peritonitis.
  2 Small/large bowel obstruction.

Peritonitis:
  1 Perforated GU, DU, ileum (complication of enteric fever) or diverticulum.
  2 Bowel infarction.
  3 Intraperitoneal haemorrhage.

Distended abdominal veins:
  1 Portal hypertension.
  2 IVC/SVC obstruction.

White or pink abdominal striae (d/t rupture of elastic fibres):
  1 Recent change in the size of abdomen (e.g. pregnancy; simple obesity;
    loss of weight; treated ascites).

Purple abdominal striae:
  1 Cushing's syndrome.

Abdominal bruising:
  1 Acute pancreatitis (→ retroperitoneal haemorrhage).
  2 Dissecting or ruptured AAA.

Palpable gallbladder:
1 Mucocoele of gallbladder.
2 Ca. gallbladder.
3 Ca. head of pancreas.

Bilateral upper abdominal masses:
1 Bilateral hydronephrosis/pyonephrosis.
2 ADPKD.
3 Amyloidosis (primary or secondary to chronic inflammation).

Unilateral mass in right or left upper quadrant:
1 Unilateral hydronephrosis/pyonephrosis; renal cyst; renal ca.
2 Distended gallbladder (on right side only).

Mass in epigastrium (±umbilical area):
1 Ca. stomach.
2 Ca. pancreas.
3 AAA.

Mass in RLQ:
1 Appendicular mass/abscess.
2 Crohn's granuloma.
3 Caecal volvulus/intussusception.
4 Ca. caecum/ascending colon.
5 Transplanted kidney.

Suprapubic mass:
1 Distended bladder.
2 Pregnant uterus.
3 Uterine fibroid/ca.
4 Ovarian cyst.

Mass in LLQ:
1 Faecal impaction.
2 Diverticular abscess.
3 Ca. descending/sigmoid colon.

Groin mass:
1 Hernia (inguinal; femoral; strangulated).
2 Lymph node (infective or malignant enlargement).
3 Cold abscess (of psoas sheath).
4 Arterial (femoral artery aneurysm).
5 Venous (saphena varix – dilatation of the long saphenous vein in the groin).

Scrotal mass:
1 Inguinal hernia descended into scrotum.
2 Testicular torsion.
3 Acute/chronic epididymo-orchitis; epididymal cyst.
4 Varicocoele (90% on the left side); spermatocoele; hydrocoele; haematocoele.
5 Tumour (seminoma; teratoma).

Enlarged prostate:
1 Prostatitis.
2 BPH.
3 Ca. prostate.

Reduced liver span (normal 12–15 cm):
1 Advanced cirrhosis.
2 Fulminant hepatitis.
3 Air under the diaphragm, e.g. secondary to rupture of a hollow viscus.

Aortic bruit:
1 Aortic narrowing (atherosclerosis); AAA; dissecting aorta.

Renal bruit:
1 Renal artery stenosis.

Hepatic bruit:
1 Hepatoma.
2 Alcoholic hepatitis.

Loin bruit:
1 Aortic narrowing (atherosclerosis); AAA; dissecting aorta.
2 Renal artery stenosis.

Central dullness, resonance in flank:
1 Distended bladder.
2 Pregnant uterus.
3 Massive ovarian cyst.

Silent abdomen (no bowel sounds):
1 Peritonitis.
2 Bowel infarction.

High-pitched bowel sounds:
1 Intestinal obstruction.
2 IBS.
3 Faecal impaction.

Intestinal obstruction:
1 Neonate/infant: congenital atresia, imperforate anus, Meckel's diverticulum, intussusception, volvulus, herniae, Hirschsprung's, meconium ileus.
2 Young/middle age adults: herniae, adhesions, Crohn's.
3 Elderly: herniae, adhesions, diverticulitis, colorectal ca., faecal impaction.

Epigastric pain:
1 Gastric causes (gastritis; peptic ulcer; worm infestation; ca. stomach).
2 Gallbladder and liver causes (cholecystitis; hepatitis).
3 Pancreatic causes (acute/chronic pancreatitis; ca. pancreas).
4 Oesophageal causes (oesophagitis).
5 Thoracic causes (MI; basal pleuritis; basal pneumonia).
6 Uncommonly, d/t small bowel infarction, ruptured or dissecting AAA.

RUQ pain:
1 Gallbladder pathology (biliary colic; cholecystitis).
2 Liver pathology (hepatitis; acute liver congestion).
3 Renal pathology (renal stones; pyelonephritis).

LUQ pain:
1 Splenic pathology (infarct; rupture).
2 Renal pathology (renal stones; pyelonephritis).

Loin pain (left or right):
1 Renal/ureteric colic (colicky pain radiating from loin to groin) d/t renal/ureteric calculi, or pyelonephritis.
2 Ruptured or dissecting AAA.

LIF pain:
1 Constipation.
2 Diverticular disease.
3 IBS.
4 IBD.
5 Pelvic referred pain (salpingitis; ectopic pregnancy; twisted/ruptured ovarian cyst, etc).
6 Ureteric colic.

RIF pain:
1 Appendicitis.
2 Mesenteric adenitis.
3 IBD.
4 Pelvic referred pain (salpingitis; ectopic pregnancy; twisted/ruptured ovarian cyst, etc).
5 Ureteric colic.

Generalised abdominal pain:
1 Generalised peritonitis.
2 Gastroenteritis.
3 Constipation.
4 IBS.

Acute central (periumbilical) abdominal pain:
1 Intestinal problem (small bowel obstruction; Crohn's disease).
2 Vascular problem (mesenteric artery occlusion [often an old patient with vascular disease]; abdominal aortic dissection).
3 Pancreatitis.

Acute lower central (hypogastric) abdominal pain:
1 UTI (cystitis).
2 Acute bladder distension (d/t BPH in males).
3 Intestinal pathology (large bowel obstruction; infective colitis/ulcerative colitis).
4 Gynaecologic pathology (ectopic pregnancy; PID; pelvic endometriosis).

Pitfalls of abdominal pain:
1 Metabolic causes: diabetic ketoacidosis, porphyria, lead poisoning, hypercalcaemia, Addison's disease.
2 Atypical referred pain: MI, basal pleurisy, basal pneumonia.

Abdominal pain and neuropathy:
1 Acute intermittent porphyria.
2 Poisoning (lead; arsenic; alcohol).
3 DKA.
4 Intra-abdominal malignancy.
5 GB syndrome.
6 Vasculitis (PAN).
7 Granulomatous disease (sarcoidosis).

Abdominal pain and renal failure:
1 Henoch–Schönlein's purpura.
2 HUS.
3 PAN.
4 Renal pathology (ADPKD; renal stones; analgesic nephropathy).
5 Acute pancreatitis.
6 Dissecting aortic aneurysm.
7 Retroperitoneal fibrosis.
8 Legionnaires' disease.
9 Ethylene glycol poisoning.

Severe weight loss over weeks or months:
1 Any advanced malignancy.
2 Chronic infection, e.g. TB.
3 Endocrine pathology (uncontrolled DM; thyrotoxicosis; Addison's disease).
4 Depression.

Vomiting:
- Vomiting **with weight loss**.
- Vomiting **without weight loss**.
- Vomiting shortly after (within hours) **food intake**.
- Vomiting unrelated to food but with **abdominal pain and fever**.
- Vomiting with **abdominal pain alone** (unrelated to food and no fever) – **non-metabolic** causes.
- Vomiting with **abdominal pain alone** (unrelated to food and no fever) – **metabolic** causes.
- Vomiting with **headache alone** (unrelated to food and no abdominal pain).
- **Vomiting alone** (unrelated to food and without abdominal pain or headache).

Vomiting with weight loss:
1 GI malignancy (oesophageal/gastric/small intestinal – lymphoma).
2 Non-malignant oesophageal pathology (oesophageal stricture; achalasia).

Vomiting without weight loss:
1 Oesophageal pathology (oesophagitis; achalasia; pharyngeal pouch).

Vomiting shortly after (within hours) food intake:
1 Gastric pathology (gastritis; GU; DU; gastric outlet obstruction d/t ca./lymphoma/peptic ulcer healing with excessive fibrosis/pyloric stenosis in the newborn; gastroparesis d/t DM).
2 Small intestinal tumour (lymphoma).
3 Acute cholecystitis (d/t cholelithiasis).
4 Acute pancreatitis.

Vomiting unrelated to food but with abdominal pain and fever:
1 Food poisoning.
2 Abdominal/pelvic infection (hepatitis A or B; acute appendicitis/mesenteric adenitis; malaria; GE; UTI; pelvic inflammatory disease; toxic shock syndrome secondary to tampon use).
3 Chest infection (lower-lobe pneumonia).
4 Haemolytic uraemic syndrome (HUS).

Vomiting with abdominal pain alone (unrelated to food and no fever) – non-metabolic causes:

1 Large bowel obstruction (d/t malignancy; strangulated hernia; intussusception).
2 Mesenteric artery occlusion.
3 Hepatic ca. (secondary or primary).
4 Renal stones.
5 Gynaecologic causes (ectopic pregnancy; miscarriage).
6 Heart pathology (acute inferior wall MI; CCF → hepatic congestion).

Vomiting with abdominal pain alone (unrelated to food and no fever) – metabolic causes:

1 Drug overdosage (e.g. digoxin toxicity).
2 DKA.
3 Acute intermittent porphyria.
4 Hypercalcaemia.
5 Lead poisoning/vitamin A intoxication.
6 Phaeochromocytoma.

Vomiting with headache alone (unrelated to food and no abdominal pain):

1 CNS pathology (migraine; meningitis; severe hypertension; haemorrhagic stroke; ↑ ICP; epilepsy).
2 Eye pathology (acute glaucoma).
3 Endocrine pathology (Addison's disease).

Vomiting alone (unrelated to food and without abdominal pain or headache):

1 Anaphylaxis.
2 ENT pathology (acute viral labyrinthitis; Ménière's disease).
3 GI pathology (sliding hiatus hernia; GE).
4 Pregnancy.
5 CRF.
6 Addison's disease.
7 Drugs (e.g. antibiotics; cytotoxics; any overdosage; excessive alcohol intake).
8 Functional.

Sore throat:

1 Acute pharyngitis.
2 Acute follicular tonsillitis (streptococcal).
3 Meningococcal meningitis.
4 Infectious mononucleosis (glandular fever) d/t Epstein–Barr virus.
5 Candidiasis of buccal or oesophageal mucosa.
6 Agranulocytosis.

Dysphagia:
1 Oropharyngeal pathology (stomatitis; tonsillitis; pharyngitis).
2 GORD.
3 Stricture (benign; malignant).
4 Motility disorder (achalasia; scleroderma; diffuse oesophageal spasm – intermittent).
5 Paralysis of the pharyngeal muscles (bulbar/pseudobulbar palsy; myasthenia gravis; dermatomyositis; polymyositis; oculo-pharyngeal myopathy).
6 Plummer–Vinson's syndrome.
7 Infectious oesophagitis (HSV; candida).
8 Exogenous compression of oesophagus (retrosternal thyroid; thymoma; enlarged mediastinal lymph nodes d/t lymphoma, leukaemia, metastases; enlarged left atrium d/t MS).
9 Globus hystericus.

Dysphagia for solids which stick:
1 Stricture (benign; malignant – ca. oesophagus/gastric cardia).
2 Exogenous oesophageal compression.

Dysphagia (solids > fluids) – no 'sticking' of the solids:
1 Xerostomia.
2 Pharyngeal pouch/pharyngo-oesophageal diverticulum.
3 Postcricoid web (congenital or Plummer-Vinson's syndrome).
4 Globus pharyngeus.

Dysphagia (fluids > solids):
1 Motility disorder (achalasia; scleroderma; diffuse oesophageal spasm – intermittent).
2 Paralysis of the pharyngeal muscles (bulbar/pseudobulbar palsy; myasthenia gravis; dermatomyositis; polymyositis).

Persistent/recurrent vomiting:
1 CRF.
2 Oesophageal obstruction (d/t achalasia); gastric outlet obstruction (d/t ca. stomach; chronic DU; post gastric surgery); intestinal obstruction.
3 Pregnancy.
4 ↑ ICP (head injury; SOL, e.g. haematoma, abscess, tumour; cyst; AVM; meningitis; encephalitis).
5 Labyrinthine disorders (vestibular neuronitis; Ménière's disease; acoustic neuroma; drugs, e.g. streptomycin, furosemide; quinine; salicylates).
6 Psychogenic.

Haematemesis/melaena:
1 Gastric disease (peptic ulcer; erosive gastritis; ca. stomach).

2 Oesophageal disease (erosive oesophagitis; oesophageal varices; ca. oesophagus).
3 Mallory–Weiss' syndrome.
4 Ingestion of corrosives.
5 False haematemesis: swallowing of nose bleed or haemoptysis.
6 Rarely (hereditary haemorrhagic telangiectasia; bleeding disorder).

Gastritis:
1 *Helicobacter pylori.*
2 Drugs (NSAIDs; aspirin; KCl; theophylline).
3 Stress (head injury; burns; shock/sepsis; hepatic encephalopathy; uraemic gastritis).
4 Atrophic gastritis (pernicious anaemia).

Jejunal villous atrophy:
1 Coeliac disease.
2 Whipple's disease.
3 Tropical sprue.
4 Hypogammaglobulinaemia.
5 Lymphoma.

Protein-losing enteropathy:
Gastric pathology:
1 Ménétrier's disease (giant hypertrophy of gastric rugae).
2 Gastric carcinoma.

Intestinal pathology:
1 IBD.
2 Whipple's disease.
3 Tropical sprue.
4 Hypogammaglobulinaemia.
5 Intestinal lymphangiectasia.

Skin pathology:
1 Erythroderma.

Acute intestinal pseudo-obstruction:
1 Postoperative.
2 Electrolyte disturbance (hypokalaemia; hyper- or hypocalcaemia; hypomagnesaemia).
3 Hypothyroidism.
4 Liver failure.
5 Acute pancreatitis.
6 Acute cholecystitis.

7 Intestinal ischaemia.
8 Retroperitoneal haematoma.

Chronic intestinal pseudo-obstruction:
Neurological:
1 DM.
2 Chagas' disease.
3 Parkinsonism.

Myopathy:
1 Polymyositis.
2 Dystrophia myotonica.

Muscle infiltration:
1 Amyloidosis.
2 Systemic sclerosis.

Other intestinal disorders:
1 Coeliac disease.
2 Jejunal diverticulosis.

Drug-induced:
1 CVS drugs (anticholinergics; Ca^{2+} antagonists).
2 CNS drugs (opiates; antidepressants; phenothiazines).
3 Iron.

Bleeding per rectum:
1 Anal pathology (haemorrhoids; anal fissure; fistula-in-ano).
2 Tumour (colorectal ca.; precancerous polyps).
3 IBD.
4 Diverticulitis.
5 Non-accidental trauma/sexual assault (especially in children).
6 Rarely (Meckel's diverticulum; intussusception; ischaemic colitis; mesenteric infarction; rapid transit of upper GI bleed; AVM; bleeding disorder).

Acute (<2 weeks duration) non-bloody/watery diarrhoea:
1 Food poisoning.[1]
2 Infection:
   a   Viral (rotavirus; norovirus; adenovirus).

---

[1] Causes other than bacterial infection, e.g. allergy to certain foods (e.g. shellfish, unripe fruit); chemical poisons (e.g. arsenic); bacterial toxins (e.g. enterotoxigenic *E. coli*; *S. aureus*; *Clostridium perfringens/botulinum*).

  b Protozoal (giardiasis).
  c Bacterial (traveller's diarrhoea d/t enterotoxigenic *Escherichia. coli* or *Shigella*; *Vibrio cholerae*).
3 Spurious diarrhoea (secondary to faecal impaction).

Acute bloody diarrhoea:
1 Food poisoning.[2]
2 Dysentery (amoebic/bacillary[3]).
3 IBD (first attack).
4 Colitis:
  a Pseudomembranous colitis (*Clostridium difficile* infection secondary to antibiotic therapy with ampicillin, clindamycin, etc).
  b Ischaemic colitis.
  c *Yersinia enterocolitica* colitis.

Sudden diarrhoea, fever and vomiting:
1 Food poisoning/toxins:
  a Eating doubtful **meat**: *Staphylococcus aureus* (incubation period <6 hr), *Salmonella typhimurium*, *Clostridium perfringens* (incubation period 8–16 hr).
  b Eating doubtful **seafood**: *Vibrio parahaemolyticus* (incubation period 16–72 hr).
  c Eating doubtful **canned food:** botulism (incubation period 18–36 hr).
  d Eating doubtful **rice**: *Bacillus cereus* (incubation period <6 hr).
2 Viral gastroenteritis: rotavirus (<5-yr-olds; resolves within a week) and norovirus (>5-yr-olds and adults; resolves in two weeks).
3 Pseudomembranous colitis.

Chronic (>4 weeks duration) non-bloody diarrhoea:
1 Malabsorption (coeliac disease; Whipple's disease; tropical sprue; lactase deficiency; chronic pancreatitis; gastric/intestinal resection); bacterial colonisation of small bowel (d/t blind loops after surgery; diverticulosis; stricture/fistula formation secondary to Crohn's disease).
2 Intestinal TB/Crohn's disease/IBS/giardiasis/HIV infection.
3 Diabetic diarrhoea.
4 Thyrotoxicosis.
5 Laxative abuse; antibiotics; antihypertensives; alcohol.
6 Faecal impaction with overflow.
7 Zollinger-Ellison's syndrome.

---

2 Bacterial infections, e.g. enterohaemorrhagic *E. coli*; *Campylobacter jejuni*; *Salmonella typhimurium*.
3 D/t *Shigella dysenteriae/flexneri/boydii/sonnei*.

8 Carcinoid syndrome.

Chronic bloody diarrhoea:
1 Recurrent amoebic dysentery.
2 IBD.
3 Colorectal ca.

Diarrhoea alternating with constipation:
1 Intestinal TB.
2 IBS.
3 Chronic amoebic dysentery.
4 Colorectal ca.

Complications of ulcerative colitis:
1 Haemorrhage.
2 Toxic megacolon.[4]
3 Colonic perforation.
4 Septicaemia.
5 Ca. colon (in longstanding cases).

Complications of Crohn's Disease:
1 Malabsorption (especially vitamin B_{12}).
2 Stricture formation ($\rightarrow$ intestinal obstruction).
3 Abscess.
4 Fistulas (enterocutaneous; ileocolic; ileovesical; perianal).
5 Haemorrhage.
6 Perforation.

Extraintestinal manifestations of ulcerative colitis:
1 Clubbing of fingers.
2 Eye (episcleritis; iridocyclitis).
3 Cholangitis.
4 Pyoderma gangrenosum.
5 Enteropathic arthritis.

Chronic constipation:
1 Diet and life style (low fibre/low fluid intake; sedentary).
2 Persistent and intentional suppression of the urge to defaecate/poor bowel training.
3 Hypothyroidism.

---

4   Presents with abdominal pain, tenderness, distension with associated high swinging fever and tachycardia. Plain X-ray abdomen will show dilated colon (transverse colon diameter >5 cm with loss of haustrations).

4 Irritable bowel syndrome.

5 Drugs (opioids; anticholinergics; tricyclics; aluminium-containing antacids; diuretics).

6 Hypercalcaemia.

7 Autonomic neuropathy (d/t DM; acute intermittent porphyria; lead poisoning).

8 Megacolon (Hirschsprung's disease; complication of ulcerative colitis).

Acute/recent onset constipation:
1 Painful anorectal lesions (fissure-in-ano; fistula-in-ano).

2 Intestinal obstruction.

3 Paralytic ileus.

4 Acute illness (↓ fluid and food intake → constipation).

5 Colorectal carcinoma.

Tenesmus (intense desire to defaecate but no stools):
1 Rectal pathology (inflammation – proctitis; colorectal ca.).

2 PID.

Anorectal pain:
1 Anal/peri-anal pathology (proctitis; fissure-in-ano; thrombotic haemorrhoids; peri-anal abscess).

2 Prostatic pathology (prostatitis).

3 Proctalgia fugax/coccydynia (rectal or coccygeal pain related to sitting and not defaecation + tenderness of levator muscle on physical examination).

Urinary frequency ± dysuria:
1 UTI.

2 BPH.

3 Bladder/urethral calculus; spastic bladder d/t UMN lesion.

4 Uterine prolapse.

Pre-hepatic jaundice:
1 Haemolysis (haemoglobinopathies, e.g. sickle-cell anaemia, thalassaemia; congenital spherocytosis; G6PD deficiency; malaria; antibody-related haemolysis like incompatible blood transfusion, septicaemia, etc).

2 Ineffective erythropoiesis d/t vitamin B_{12}/folic acid deficiency.

Hepatic jaundice:
1 Hepatitis.
  a Viral (A, B, C, D, E).
  b Alcoholic.[5]

---

5   Alcoholic liver diseases include fatty liver; alcoholic hepatitis; cirrhosis.

  c Autoimmune.

  d Drugs (dose-related [e.g. PCM, tetracycline]; idiosyncratic [antituberculous, e.g. rifampicin, INH, pyrazinamide; chlorpromazine; halothane]).

2 Malignancy (metastases; HCC).

3 Right heart failure.

4 Pregnancy-related jaundice (acute fatty liver of pregnancy; recurrent intrahepatic cholestasis).

5 Glandular fever (infectious mononucleosis).

6 Reye's syndrome.

7 Congenital (Gilbert's syndrome; Crigler–Najjar's syndrome; Dubin–Johnson's syndrome; Rotor's syndrome).

Post-hepatic (obstructive) jaundice:

1 Stones in the CBD (choledocholithiasis).

2 Stricture of the CBD (benign [usually iatrogenic]; malignant [primary cholangiocarcinoma]).

3 Distal CBD obstruction (chronic pancreatitis; ca. head of pancreas; ca. ampulla of Vater).

4 Enlarged lymph nodes at porta hepatis (usually malignant enlargement).

5 Pregnancy (3rd trimester).

Other causes of obstructive jaundice/cholestasis:

1 Sepsis.

2 Hepatitis/cirrhosis.

3 PSC; PBC.

4 Dubin–Johnson's syndrome ($\downarrow$ excretion of conjugated bilirubin).

5 Drug-induced cholestasis (OCPs; erythromycin; flucloxacillin; anabolic steroids; phenothiazines).

6 Total parenteral nutrition (TPN).

Unconjugated hyperbilirubinaemia:

1 Haemolysis (haemoglobinopathies, e.g. sickle-cell anaemia, thalassaemia; congenital spherocytosis; G6PD deficiency; malaria; antibody-related haemolysis, e.g. incompatible blood transfusion).

2 Ineffective erythropoiesis (B_{12}/folate deficiency).

3 Neonatal physiological jaundice.

4 Congenital (Gilbert's syndrome; Crigler–Najjar's syndrome).

HBV – markers of replicative phase (high infectivity):

1 Positive: HBsAg, HBeAg, HBcAg in hepatocytes and HBV DNA.

2 Negative: anti-HBe

HBV – markers of non-replicative phase (low infectivity):
1 Positive: HBsAg and anti-HBe.
2 Negative: HBeAg, HBcAg in hepatocytes and HBV DNA.

Autoimmune hepatitis – associated disorders:
1 Haemolytic anaemia (Coomb's positive).
2 Thyroid pathology (thyrotoxicosis; myxoedema; thyroiditis).
3 Lymphadenopathy.
4 Pleurisy.
5 Pleural infiltration.
6 Ulcerative colitis.
7 Glomerulonephritis.
8 Polyarthritis.

Viral hepatic markers – interpretation:
- IgM anti-HAV: acute hepatitis A.
- IgG anti-HAV: immune to hepatitis A (d/t previous infection).
- HBsAg (Australia antigen):
  - Acute hepatitis B.
  - Chronic hepatitis B.
  - Carrier state.
- HBsAg + anti-HBe + absent HBeAg: virus is present but not actively replicating.
- HBsAg + HBV DNA + absent HBeAg: pre-core mutant virus is present.
- HBeAg: virus is actively replicating, the disease is active and the patient highly infectious.
- HBV DNA: more-direct evidence of replicating virus than HBeAg – positive even in mutant virus.
- Anti-HBs: immune to hepatitis B.
- HBsAg and anti-HBs are both negative: non-immune subject ($\rightarrow$ vaccinate).
- HBsAg negative and anti-HBs positive: immune subject (no need to vaccinate).
- HBsAg positive + both HBeAg and anti-HBe negative: healthy carrier (no need to vaccinate).
- IgM anti-HBc: acute hepatitis B.
- HBeAg + IgM anti-HBc: acute hepatitis B.
- HBeAg + IgG anti-HBc: chronic hepatitis B.
- HBsAg + IgG anti-HBc: chronic hepatitis B.
- IgG anti-HBc with negative HBsAg: past exposure to hepatitis B.
- HCV RNA: actively replicating HCV.
- Anti-HCV: acute or chronic hepatitis C.
- HDV Ag: acute hepatitis D.

- IgM anti-HDV: acute hepatitis D.
- IgG anti-HDV: past HDV infection.
- Anti-HEV: acute hepatitis E.

HBsAg – related issues:
1 Whether it is a case of acute or chronic hepatitis B.
2 Whether the virus is in the replicative or non-replicative phase.[6]
3 Whether or not co-infection with HDV present.

Acute hepatitis – viral markers:
1 Acute hepatitis A: IgM anti-HAV.
2 Acute hepatitis A + hepatitis B carrier: IgM anti-HAV + HBsAg.
3 Acute hepatitis B: HBsAg + IgM anti-HBc.[7]
4 Acute hepatitis C: HCV RNA (within 2 weeks) + anti-HCV (after 2–3 months).
5 Acute hepatitis D: HBsAg + IgM anti-HDV.
6 Acute hepatitis E: IgM anti-HEV.

Chronic hepatitis – viral markers:
1 Chronic hepatitis B (replicative phase): HBsAg + IgG HBcAg + HBeAg + HBV DNA.
2 Chronic hepatitis B (non-replicative phase): HBsAg and IgG HBcAg are positive; HBeAg and HBV DNA are negative.
3 Chronic hepatitis C: HCV RNA + anti-HCV.
4 Past exposure to HCV: HCV RNA negative; anti-HCV positive.

Indications for hepatitis B vaccination:
1 Doctors; paramedical staff.
2 Spouse/children of a HBsAg-positive person.
3 Baby born to a HBsAg-positive mother.
4 Universal immunisation as part of the EPI program.

Complications of hepatitis B:
1 Acute fulminant hepatic failure.
2 Chronic active hepatitis.
3 Cirrhosis.
4 Hepatocellular ca.

Exudative ascites (protein >2.5 g/dL or serum-ascites albumin gradient <1.1):
1 Infection (tuberculous peritonitis; bacterial peritonitis).

---

6   Non-replicative phase practically means a carrier state.

7   Presence of IgM anti-HBc means acute hepatitis B even if HBsAg is negative.

2 Malignant dissemination.
3 Chemical peritonitis (as occurs in peptic ulcer perforation secondary to HCl or bile).
4 Acute pancreatitis.

Transudative ascites (protein <2.5 g/dL or serum-ascites albumin gradient >1.1):
1 Liver disease (cirrhosis).
2 Congestion (right heart failure; constrictive pericarditis; pericardial effusion; inferior vena cava obstruction; Budd–Chiari's syndrome, i.e. hepatic veins obstruction).
3 Hypoproteinaemia (nephrotic syndrome; starvation; protein-losing enteropathy, etc).
4 Meigs' syndrome.

Acute fulminant hepatic failure:
1 Drug overdosage (PCM; tetracycline).
2 Toxins (carbon tetrachloride).
3 Viral hepatitis (especially HBV).
4 Acute fatty liver of pregnancy.
5 Reye's syndrome.

Features of cerebral oedema in acute fulminant hepatic failure:
1 Eyes: disconjugate eye movements; abnormal pupillary response.
2 Respiration: hyperventilation.
3 Motor: decerebrate rigidity; focal fits.

Bad prognostic signs in acute fulminant hepatic failure:
(four clinical and six lab):

Clinical:
1 Age <11 or >40 yrs.
2 Duration of jaundice before encephalopathy >7 days.
3 Small liver.
4 Ascites.

Lab:
1 Serum bilirubin >18 mg/dL.
2 PT >50 sec.
3 Serum albumin <3.5 g/dL.
4 Factor V <15%.
5 Persistent hypoglycaemia.
6 EEG showing triphasic waves.

Cirrhosis of liver:
1 Alcohol.
2 Chronic hepatitis (chronic viral hepatitis B and C; autoimmune [lupoid] hepatitis).
3 Drugs (α-methyldopa; methotrexate, etc).
4 Metabolic disease (haemochromatosis;[8] Wilson's disease; α1-antitrypsin deficiency).
5 Congestion/cholestasis (congestion d/t right heart failure; cholestasis d/t PBC, prolonged extrahepatic obstruction secondary to any cause, etc).

Complications of cirrhosis:
1 Ascites.
2 Spontaneous peritonitis.
3 Variceal bleed.
4 Hepatoma.
5 Hepatorenal syndrome.
6 Hepatic encephalopathy.

Precipitating factors for encephalopathy in a cirrhotic:
1 GIT: GI bleeding; $\uparrow$ protein diet; constipation.
2 Ascitic fluid: excessive paracentesis; excessive diuresis; SBP.
3 Electrolytes: $\downarrow$ K$^+$.
4 Drugs: sedatives; diuretics.
5 Trauma/surgery.

Hepatic cirrhosis + dilated cardiomyopathy:
1 Alcoholism.
2 Haemochromatosis.

Hepatic granulomas + restrictive cardiomyopathy:
1 Sarcoidosis.

Hepatic dysfunction + cardiomyopathy:
1 Storage disorders.

Hepatic congestion + right heart failure:
1 Right heart failure/CCF.
2 Constrictive pericarditis.
3 Pericardial effusion.
4 Tricuspid regurgitation.
5 IVC obstruction.

---

8   D/t: primary; secondary (chronic haemolytic anaemia; sideroblastic anaemia; multiple blood transfusions).

6 Budd–Chiari's syndrome.

Budd–Chiari's syndrome (hepatic veins obstruction):
1 Luminal obstruction (thrombosis [d/t OCPs, polycythaemia vera]; congenital web).
2 Exogenous infiltration (invasion by a tumour – hepatic, renal, adrenal, gastric, pancreatic).

Hepatomegaly:
1 Acute/chronic hepatitis (viral, alcohol- or drug-induced); cirrhosis.
2 Congestive hepatomegaly (right heart failure, etc).
3 Infection (amoebic/pyogenic abscess; hydatid cyst; typhoid fever; miliary tuberculosis; infectious mononucleosis; septicaemia).
4 Malignancy (metastases; lymphoma; leukaemia; HCC).
5 Metabolic disorders (DM; haemochromatosis; glycogen-storage diseases).
6 Healthy person (Riedel's lobe and prominent left lobe).

Hepatomegaly – smooth and tender:
1 Acute hepatitis (viral, alcohol- or drug-induced).
2 Congestive hepatomegaly (right heart failure d/t tricuspid regurgitation or acute pulmonary hypertension secondary to pulmonary embolism).
3 Infection (amoebic/pyogenic abscess; hydatid cyst; typhoid fever; miliary tuberculosis; infectious mononucleosis; septicaemia).

Hepatomegaly – smooth and non-tender:
1 Cirrhosis of liver; primary biliary cirrhosis.
2 Amyloidosis (primary or secondary to chronic inflammation).
3 Metabolic disease (haemochromatosis).
4 Malignancy (lymphoma; leukaemia).

Hepatomegaly – irregular, non-tender:
1 Malignancy (metastases; HCC).
2 Hydatid cyst.

Hepatocellular carcinoma (HCC):
1 Cirrhosis d/t any cause.
2 Aflatoxin (produced by *Aspergillus flavus* – it contaminates foodstuffs especially corn and peanuts stored in warm and damp conditions).

Hepatic metastases + pericardial effusion:
1 Neoplasia.

Hepatic metastases + PS/TS:
1 Carcinoid syndrome (with hepatic metastases).

Hepatitis + pericarditis:
1 HIV.

Splenomegaly:
1 Infection (viral hepatitis – A, B, C or D; malaria; typhoid fever; miliary TB; infective endocarditis; infectious mononucleosis; brucella; leishmaniasis).
2 Portal hypertension (usually secondary to cirrhosis of liver).
3 Haemolytic anaemia.
4 Connective tissue disorder (SLE, etc.).
5 Amyloidosis (primary or secondary to chronic inflammation).
6 Malignancy (lymphoma; leukaemia; myeloproliferative disorders).

Splenomegaly – slight (<3 fingers):
1 Infection (viral hepatitis – A, B, C or D; malaria; typhoid fever; miliary TB; infective endocarditis; infectious mononucleosis; brucella; leishmaniasis).
2 Haemolytic anaemia.
3 Connective tissue disorder (SLE, etc.).
4 Amyloidosis (primary or secondary to chronic inflammation).

Splenomegaly – moderate (3–5 fingers):
1 Portal hypertension (usually secondary to cirrhosis of liver).
2 Malignancy (lymphoma; leukaemia).

Massive splenomegaly (>5 fingers/>8 cm below LCM and/or weight >1 kg):
1 Infection (chronic malaria; leishmaniasis).
2 CML.
3 Myelofibrosis.
4 Polycythaemia vera.

Differentiation between CML and myelofibrosis:
1 Massive splenomegaly with very high TLC ($>50 \times 10^9/L$) is found in both.
2 Peripheral blood film in CML shows numerous granulocytes at varying stages of maturation; in myelofibrosis teardrop cells are seen; leucoerythroblastic picture can be found in both.
3 Bone marrow biopsy will show numerous granulocytes at varying stages of maturation in CML; diffuse fibrosis is seen in myelofibrosis (stains black with reticulin).
4 Whereas leucocyte alkaline phosphatase is low in CML, it is either normal or high in myelofibrosis.
5 Philadelphia chromosome is present only in CML cases (90%).

Hepatosplenomegaly:
1 Infection (acute/chronic hepatitis, infectious mononucleosis).
2 Cirrhosis of liver; portal hypertension.
3 Malignancy (leukaemia; lymphoma).
4 Enteric fever.
5 β-thalassaemia.
6 Glycogen-storage disease.

Acute pancreatitis:
1 Gallstones.
2 Alcohol.
3 ERCP.
4 Abdominal trauma.
5 Fulminant hepatic failure.
6 Hyperlipidaemia.
7 Hypercalcaemia.

Acute pancreatitis – complications:
1 Pancreatic necrosis, phlegmon, abscess, pseudocyst.
2 Shock ($\rightarrow$ renal failure).
3 Gastric erosions ($\rightarrow$ haematemesis).
4 ARDS.

↑ Amylase:
1 Acute pancreatitis and its complications.
2 ERCP.
3 Cholangitis/cholecystitis.
4 Acute/chronic liver pathology.
5 Salpingitis/ectopic pregnancy/ovarian tumour.
6 End-stage renal disease.
7 Salivary adenitis.

Acalculous cholecystitis:
1 Diabetes mellitus.
2 Severe trauma, burns, major surgery, etc.

6 Neurology

Extrapyramidal system (concerned with movements and posture) consists of:
1 Basal ganglia.
2 Substantia nigra.
3 Subthalamic nuclei.
4 Red nuclei.

Posture:
1 Decorticate posture:[1]
  a Severe bilateral damage to the hemisphere above the midbrain.
2 Decerebrate posture:[2]
  a Damage to the midbrain (diencephalon).

Formulae to determine which spinal segment lies against a particular vertebral body:
- For cervical vertebra: add 1 (e.g. against 5th cervical vertebra, there will be (5+1) 6th cervical spinal segment).
- For T1–T6: add 2.
- For T7–T9: add 3.
- T10: lies over L1 and L2.
- T11: lies over L3 and L4.
- T12: lies over L5 and upper sacral segments.
- L1: lies over lower sacral and coccygeal spinal segments.

Internal capsule blood supply:
1 Lenticulostriate arteries (branches of middle cerebral artery).
2 Heubner's artery (branch of anterior cerebral artery) – supplies fibres concerned with face and upper limb.

Grasp reflex:
1 Contralateral frontal lobe lesion.

---

1 Spontaneous flexion of elbow and wrist joints + supination of the arm + extension of the legs.
2 Spontaneous extension of elbow and wrist joints + pronation of the arm + extension of the legs.

Avoiding response:
1 Contralateral parietal lobe lesion.

Palmo-mental reflex:
1 Brain damage.

Snout reflex:
1 Bilateral UMN lesion.

Glabellar tap reflex:
1 Parkinsonism.
2 Senile dementia.

Dyslexia (inability to read):
1 Dominant parietal lobe lesion.

Dysgraphia (inability to write):
1 Frontal/parietal lobe lesion.

Speech disturbance:
Could be d/t disturbance of hearing (deafness), poor attention, receptive dysphasia, motor dysphasia, dysarthria, dysphonia or a combination of these:
1 Deafness (d/t ear disease or 8th nerve lesion) – look for features of ear disease.
2 Inattention (d/t depression or dementia).
3 Receptive dysphasia (d/t lesion in the Wernicke's area in the dominant temporal lobe).
4 Motor dysphasia (d/t lesion in the dominant frontoparietal lobe).
5 Dysarthria (d/t cerebellar, UMN/LMN lesion) – look for associated weakness/incoordination of oral muscles.
6 Dysphonia (d/t vocal cord paralysis) – confirm on indirect laryngoscopy.

Dysarthria:
1 Cerebral cortical lesion (dysarthria + other cortical signs).
2 Internal capsule lesion (dysarthria + other internal capsule signs, e.g. spastic hemiparesis).
3 Pseudobulbar palsy – UMN lesion (dysarthria 'nasal quality speech' + dysphagia + spastic hemiparesis).
4 Bulbar palsy – LMN lesion (dysarthria 'nasal quality speech – Donald Duck quality speech' + dysphagia + spastic hemiparesis).
5 Extrapyramidal dysarthria (d/t parkinsonism) – difficulty initiating speech, which is slow + other signs of parkinsonism.
6 Cerebellar lesion d/t ischaemia, SOL, MS, hereditary ataxia (scanning speech + other cerebellar signs).

7 Drugs, e.g. alcohol/sedatives (dysarthria + other drug effects).

Scanning speech:
1 Cerebellar dysfunction.

Slurring speech:
1 Bulbar palsy.
2 Pseudobulbar (supranuclear) palsy.

Dysphonia (change in the quality of voice or loss of volume of voice):
1 Laryngitis.
2 Vocal cord paralysis – 10th nerve palsy.

Aphonia (complete loss of voice):
1 Hysteria (commonest cause).
2 Bilateral vocal cord paralysis.

Bradylalia (unduly slow speech):
1 Myxoedema.

Echolalia (subject automatically repeats examiner's questions):
1 Normal (in early childhood).
2 Widespread brain damage.

Palilalia (subject repeats last sentence/phrase/word of his own speech):
1 Extensive cerebrovascular disease.
2 Postencephalitis parkinsonism.

Anosmia:
1 Nasal pathology (coryza, i.e. common cold; nasal allergy).
2 Head injury → skull fracture.
3 Tuberculous meningitis.
4 Tumour of anterior cranial fossa.
5 Kallman's syndrome (anosmia + delayed puberty/poor secondary sexual characteristics/infertility/primary amenorrhoea in females + ↓ FSH, LH, testosterone or oestrogen).

Parosmia (perversion of smell – offensive smells are perceived as pleasant smells and vice versa):
1 Psychogenic.

Hallucinations of smell:
1 Temporal lobe epilepsy.

Optic atrophy (pale optic disc):
1 Primary (pale disc with well-defined margins).
2 Secondary to longstanding papilloedema (pale disc with irregular and blurred margins).

Papilloedema – diagnostic features:
1 Red, swollen disc with obliteration of physiological cup and blurred margins (nasal margin first).
2 Engorged retinal veins.
3 Loss of pulsations of retinal veins.
4 Small haemorrhages.
5 **Normal visual acuity**.

Papillitis – diagnostic features:
1 Changes are similar to those of papilloedema. Distinction between the two is made on the basis of visual acuity. Whereas, in papillitis, there occurs marked deterioration of the vision, in papilloedema, visual acuity remains normal except for an enlargement of the blind spot.

Visual field defects:
1 Complete loss of vision:
   a Lesion of the optic nerve.
2 Central scotoma:
   a Ipsilateral optic nerve disease (optic neuritis, etc).
3 Bitemporal hemianopia:
   a Optic chiasmal lesion:
      i Tumour (pituitary; craniopharyngioma; meningioma).
      ii Anterior communicating artery aneurysm.
      iii Dilated 3rd ventricle.
4 Homonymous hemianopia – less congruous:
   a Lesion of the contralateral optic tract.
5 Homonymous hemianopia – highly congruous:
   a Lesion of the contralateral visual cortex.
6 Homonymous hemianopia with sparing of the macula:
   a Lesion of the contralateral optic radiation in the posterior part of the parietal lobe.

Visual field defects – underlying aetiology:
1 Psychogenic (normal VA, colour vision, optic disc).
2 Retinitis pigmentosa.
3 Chorioretinitis.
4 Optic chiasm lesion:
   a Tumour (pituitary; craniopharyngioma; suprasellar meningioma).
   b Anterior communicating artery aneurysm.

   c Dilated 3rd ventricle.
5 Optic tract lesion:
   a Middle cerebral artery occlusion of contralateral side.
   b Tumour/SOL.
6 Visual cortex lesion:
   a Posterior cerebral artery occlusion of contralateral side.
   b Tumour/SOL.

Chorioretinitis:
1 Infection (HIV; CMV; toxoplasmosis; toxocariasis; syphilis).
2 Granulomatous disease (TB; sarcoidosis).
3 Behçet's syndrome.
4 Trauma.

3rd nerve palsy:
1 DM (painful eye movements; pupils remain unaffected).
2 Pituitary tumour/meningioma.
3 Cavernous sinus thrombosis/intracavernous aneurysm (4th and 6th nerves also affected).
4 Aneurysm of the posterior communicating artery.
5 Midbrain lesion – d/t ischaemia, syphilis (ipsilateral 3rd nerve palsy with contralateral hemiplegia).

4th nerve palsy:
1 Isolated lesion is rare ($\rightarrow$ superior oblique is paralysed).

6th nerve palsy:
1 ↑ ICP d/t any cause (isolated 6th nerve palsy is referred to as false localising sign).
2 Pontine lesion → 6th and 7th nerves palsies with contralateral hemiplegia.
3 Ischaemia – diabetes.

Bilateral internuclear ophthalmoplegia:
1 Multiple sclerosis.

In cases of unilateral ophthalmoplegia, lesion is in the medial longitudinal bundle on the side of weakness of adduction.

Pupillary size:
1 Normal: 3–5 mm
2 Dilated pupil: >5 mm.
3 Constricted pupil: <3 mm.

Amblyopic light reaction (Marcus Gunn's pupil):
1 Optic nerve lesion (e.g. optic neuritis, ischaemia) → ipsilateral reduced acuity.

Direct light reflex is impaired in the affected eye, but its consensual light reflex is normal, i.e. light shone in the normal eye → normal pupillary constriction in the affected eye; if immediately afterwards, light is shone in the affected eye, pupil dilates (because direct reflex cannot maintain consensually induced constriction).

Argyll Robertson's pupil:
1 Neurosyphilis.

Lesion is in the pretectal area of midbrain.

Holmes–Adie's pupil (benign condition of no consequence):
1 Lesion is in the ciliary ganglion.

Affected pupil is larger than fellow pupil (anisocoria). Light reflex is absent (direct *and* consensual), but pupil reacts to accommodation, though the response is delayed and sustained (called tonic pupillary reaction).
 If accompanied by absent ankle jerk – called Holmes–Adie's syndrome.

Impaired vertical conjugate gaze:
1 Progressive supranuclear palsy.
2 Thyroid ophthalmopathy.
3 Myasthenia gravis.
4 Miller Fisher's syndrome.[3]

Vertigo:
1 Vestibular system disturbance (commonest cause).

Physiologic vertigo: motion/sea sickness d/t unfamiliar head movements.

Pathologic vertigo: peripheral or central pathology:

Peripheral origin:
1 Middle-ear disease (chronic otitis media ± labyrinthine fistula).
2 Inner-ear disease:
  a Vestibular neuronitis.
  b Benign paroxysmal positional vertigo (BPPV).[4]

---

3 Variant of GB syndrome – LMN type paraparesis + ophthalmoplegia.

4 Pathology is in the posterior semicircular canal.

    c Ménière's disease (recurrent peripheral vertigo + tinnitus + deafness).
3 8th nerve lesion (acoustic neuroma/schwannoma of 8th nerve): recurrent peripheral vertigo + tinnitus + deafness + 7th nerve lesion (facial weakness) + 5th nerve lesion (facial sensory loss).
4 Facial nerve disease:
    a Ramsay Hunt's syndrome.
5 Psychogenic (chronic vertigo + agoraphobia + absent nystagmus + normal CNS examination).
6 Drugs:
    a Ototoxic drugs (aminoglycosides; salicylates; phenytoin; quinine).
    b Drug toxicity (phenytoin; barbiturates; alcohol).

Central origin:
1 Brainstem ischaemia (vertebrobasilar insufficiency).
2 Cerebellar pathology.
3 Posterior fossa disease:
    a Posterior fossa tumour.
4 Cerebral disease:
    a Migraine.
    b Multiple sclerosis.
    c Temporal lobe epilepsy.
5 Mamillary body disease:
    a Wernicke's encephalopathy (d/t thiamine deficiency usually in alcoholics).

Vertigo:
Episodic with aural symptoms:
1 Ménière's disease.
2 Migraine.

Episodic without aural symptoms:
1 Benign positional vertigo.

Constant with aural symptoms:
1 Chronic otitis media with labyrinthine fistula.

Constant without aural symptoms:
1 Multiple sclerosis.

Syncope:
1 Postural syncope.
2 Vasovagal syncope.
3 Heart/vessel problem (AS; HOCM; arrhythmia – Stokes–Adams' attack; postural hypotension; carotid sinus syncope).

4 Cough/micturition syncope.
5 Exertional.
6 Hypoglycaemia.
7 Epilepsy.

Nystagmus:
1 Congenital.
2 Acquired:
    a Vestibular pathology (fast phase away from the side of the lesion).
    b Cerebellar pathology (fast phase towards the side of the lesion).
    c Drug-induced (alcohol; amitriptyline; phenytoin; phenobarbitone).

Pendular nystagmus:
1 Loss of macular vision.

Jerky nystagmus of constant direction:
1 Labyrinthine lesion.
2 Cerebellar lesion.

Nystagmus which changes its direction with the direction of the gaze:
1 Widespread central involvement of the vestibular nuclei.

Upbeat nystagmus (occurs on upwards gaze with fast component upwards):
1 Lesion in the upper part of midbrain.

Downbeat nystagmus (with fast component downwards):
1 Lesion in the lower medulla.

Trigeminal neuralgia (episodic facial pain):
1 No sign present; just pain:
    a Idiopathic (ophthalmic branch is not involved).
2 Sign/s present:
    a Postherpetic neuralgia (scarring and sensory loss over the forehead).
    b Tumour involving the 5th nerve.
    c Multiple sclerosis.

Jaw muscle weakness:
1 5th nerve palsy (UMN lesion $\rightarrow \uparrow$ jaw jerk; LMN lesion $\rightarrow \downarrow$ jaw jerk).

Facial nerve palsy:
1 Supranuclear and nuclear:
    a Cerebrovascular accident (e.g. haemorrhage or thromboembolism in the brainstem).

2 Infranuclear:
  a Bell's palsy (idiopathic facial nerve palsy) – the commonest cause.
  b Diabetes mellitus.
  c Post-traumatic (birth injury; fractured temporal bone; surgery).
  d Infection (Ramsay Hunt's syndrome [VZV infection]; ASOM; CSOM; Lyme disease).
  e Middle/inner ear pathology (otitis media; cholesteatoma; acoustic neuromas).
  f CNS pathology (stroke; multiple sclerosis; neurosarcoidosis; brainstem tumour).
  g Spinal cord pathology (GB syndrome).

Bilateral facial nerve palsy:
1 Guillain–Barré's syndrome.
2 Bulbar/pseudobulbar palsy.
3 Bilateral facial muscles weakness (myasthenia gravis; myopathy).
4 Bilateral parotid infiltration (Mikulicz's syndrome).
5 Bilateral Bell's palsy.
6 Sarcoidosis.
7 Lyme disease.

Bulbar palsy (LMN signs present – wasting of the muscles of mastication + fasciculations):
1 GB syndrome.
2 Syringobulbia.
3 Motor neuron disease (progressive muscular atrophy).
4 Bulbar polio.

Pseudobulbar palsy (UMN signs present – brisk jaw jerk):
1 Bilateral stroke.
2 Multiple sclerosis.
3 Motor neuron disease (amyotrophic lateral sclerosis; primary lateral sclerosis).

Fasciculations:
1 Motor neuron disease.
2 Spinal cord pathology (cervical spondylosis; syringomyelia; acute poliomyelitis).
3 Endocrinopathy (thyrotoxicosis).
4 Electrolyte abnormality ($\downarrow Na^+$; $\downarrow Mg^{2+}$).
5 Drug-induced (salbutamol; anticholinesterases; lithium).

Facial nerve – LMN lesion localisation:
Motor loss alone (i.e. weakness of the facial muscles alone):
  1 Lesion is after the nerve exits from the stylomastoid foramen.

Motor loss + loss of taste:
  1 Lesion is in the facial canal between the chorda tympani and branch to stapedius.

Motor loss + loss of taste + hyperacusis:
  1 Lesion is in the facial canal between the branch to stapedius and internal auditory meatus.

7th + 8th nerve palsies:
  1 Lesion is in the internal auditory meatus.

6th + 7th nerve palsies + contralateral hemiplegia:
  1 Lesion is in the pons.

5th, 6th, 7th, 8th nerve palsies and cerebellar involvement:
  1 Cerebellopontine angle tumour (facial nerve palsy + absent corneal reflex + deafness).

7th nerve palsy + vertigo + deafness:
  1 Cholesteatoma.

7th nerve palsy + vesicles over pinna (external auditory meatus):
  1 Herpes zoster infection of the geniculate ganglion (Ramsay Hunt's syndrome).

7th nerve palsy + ipsilateral midface swelling:
  1 Facial nerve palsy from parotid swelling.

Rinne's test:
  1 Air conduction is better than bone conduction (Rinne's test positive) = normal.
  2 Bone conduction is better than air conduction (Rinne's test negative) = conductive deafness.
  3 Air conduction is better than bone conduction but both are reduced (reduced positive Rinne's test) = sensorineural deafness.
  4 Bone conduction is better than air conduction but both are reduced = mixed deafness.

Weber's test:
Mnemonic: CSSO (conductive deafness same ear; sensorineural deafness opposite ear)
1 No lateralisation (equal on both sides) = test is 'central' and it indicates either normal hearing or bilaterally equal deafness.
2 Lateralised to the normal ear = sensorineural deafness.
3 Lateralised to the diseased ear = conductive deafness.

Absolute bone conduction (i.e. comparing bone conduction of the patient and doctor):
1 Doctor's bone conduction is better = patient has sensorineural deafness.
2 Equal conduction = patient has conductive deafness.

Conductive deafness:
1 External ear problem (wax [commonest cause]; foreign body; otitis externa).
2 Tympanic membrane problem (perforation secondary to trauma or acute/chronic otitis media).
3 Middle ear problem (like otitis media with effusion [OME; also called glue ear]; granuloma; otosclerosis; cholesteatoma).
4 Trauma (barotrauma; traumatic ossicular dislocation).

Sensorineural deafness:
Bilateral:
1 Commonest cause = senility (usually after 60 years of age; also called presbyacusis).
2 Trauma (noise; head injury; surgery).
3 Infection (CSOM; meningitis; measles; mumps; rubella).
4 Drugs (aminoglycosides; high-dose loop diuretics; aspirin; some β-blockers; quinine; amphotericin-B; cytotoxic drugs; lead).
5 Multiple sclerosis.
6 Ménière's disease.
7 Paget's disease.

Unilateral:
1 Cerebellopontine angle lesion (acoustic neuroma; meningioma; metastases; granuloma).

9th nerve palsy:
1 Isolated 9th nerve lesion is rare.

Recurrent laryngeal nerve (branch of 10th nerve) palsy:
1 Thyroid surgery.
2 Malignancy.

Bilateral 10th nerve palsy:
1 Bulbar and pseudobulbar palsy.
2 Jugular foramen syndrome.

11th nerve (accessory nerve) palsy:
1 Bulbar/pseudobulbar palsy (11th nerve paralysed along with other nerves).
2 Jugular foramen syndrome.

12th nerve palsy:
1 Bilateral UMN lesion – pseudobulbar palsy:
   a Tongue looks small, conical and is immobile.
2 Unilateral UMN lesion:
   a Tongue deviates towards the paralysed side on protrusion + there is no wasting.
3 Bilateral LMN lesion – bulbar palsy:
   a Bilateral wasting and fasciculations of the tongue.
4 Unilateral LMN lesion:
   a Ipsilateral wasting and fasciculations of the tongue.

Abnormal tongue, uvula and pharyngeal movement:
1 9th, 10th and 12th (not 11th) nerve lesions.

Multiple cranial nerve lesions:
1 Pituitary tumour ($\rightarrow$ optic chiasm/tract lesion; 3rd nerve lesion).
2 Anterior communicating artery aneurysm ($\rightarrow$ 2nd, 3rd and 4th nerve lesions).
3 Weber's syndrome ($\rightarrow$ ipsilateral 3rd nerve lesion and contralateral hemiparesis).
4 Posterior carotid artery aneurysm ($\rightarrow$ 4th and 5th nerve lesions).
5 Cavernous sinus lesion $\rightarrow$ 3rd, 4th, ophthalmic division of 5th and 6th nerves involved.
6 Gradenigo's syndrome (lesion in the petrous temporal bone) $\rightarrow$ 5th and 6th nerve lesions).
7 Facial canal lesions, e.g. d/t cholesteatoma ($\rightarrow$ 7th and 8th nerve lesions; **no** 5th or 6th).
8 Cerebellopontine angle tumour ($\rightarrow$ 5th, 7th and 8th ± 6th nerve lesions and cerebellar involvement).
9 Jugular foramen syndrome ($\rightarrow$ 9th, 10th and 11th nerve lesions).
10 Lateral medullary syndrome ($\rightarrow$ vertigo, Horner's syndrome, nystagmus, 5th nerve lesion, contralateral spinothalamic loss on trunk).

Head and neck muscles that push towards the opposite side:
1 Sternomastoid.

2 Genioglossus.

3 Pterygoids.

True muscle hypertrophy:

1 Body building/athletics.

2 Myotonic disorders.

Muscle pseudohypertrophy ($\uparrow$ muscle mass + $\downarrow$ power):

1 Certain muscle diseases.

Clasp-knife rigidity:

1 UMN lesion.

Lead-pipe rigidity (uniform sustained resistance throughout the range of passive movement – resembling bending a lead pipe):

1 Basal ganglia lesion.

Hysterical rigidity (resembles lead pipe rigidity though resistance increases proportionate to the amount of force applied to perform the passive movement):

1 Hysteria.

Cogwheel rigidity (tremors are superimposed on rigidity):

1 Parkinsonism.

Hypotonia:

1 LMN lesion and lesion of sensory pathways.

2 Early stages of stroke (called neuronal or spinal shock).

3 Cerebellar dysfunction.

T1 spinal segment – supplies all small muscles of the hand.

Loss of triceps jerk:

1 C7–8 posterior root lesion.

Loss of biceps jerk:

1 C5–6 posterior root lesion.

Loss of knee jerk:

1 L3–4 posterior root lesion.

Loss of ankle jerk:

1 S1–2 posterior root lesion.

Hyperreflexia in one limb or one half of the body:
1 'Contralateral' UMN cortical, internal capsule, brainstem or cervical cord lesion.
2 Cerebellar disease.

Bilaterally symmetrical hyperreflexia in all four limbs – look for the plantars:
Plantars up-going:
1 'Bilateral' UMN cortical, internal capsule, brainstem or cervical cord lesion.

Plantars down-going:
1 Anxiety.
2 Thyrotoxicosis.
3 Tetanus.

Diminished or absent reflexes:
1 LMN lesion.
2 Neuropathy (sensory[5]/motor[6]).
3 MND.
4 Poliomyelitis.
5 Tabes dorsalis.
6 Primary muscle pathology.[7]

Reflexes are usually normal in myopathies.

Deep reflexes (tendon jerks):
1 Ankle jerk.
2 Knee jerk.
3 Brachioradialis jerk.
4 Biceps jerk.
5 Triceps jerk.

Superficial reflexes:
1 Plantar reflex (S1).
2 Abdominal reflex (T8–T12).
3 Cremasteric reflex (L1–L2).
4 Anal reflex (S3–S4).
5 Conjunctival and corneal reflexes (V and VII cranial nerves).

---

5 Diminished reflexes (plantars down-going) with normal muscle power.
6 Diminished reflexes + muscle weakness, wasting and fasciculations.
7 Diminished reflexes + muscle weakness and wasting, but no fasciculations.

Absent plantar response:
1 Cold feet (repeat the test after warming the feet).
2 Paralysis of the muscles of the great toe.
3 Sensory loss over S1 dermatome.
4 Spinal shock (secondary to spinal cord transection).

Absent abdominal reflexes (T8–T12):
1 UMN lesion above T8.
2 LMN lesion involving (T8–T12).
3 Physiologically absent in obese, multiparous and old people.

Absent cremasteric reflex:
1 UMN lesion.

Romberg's sign:
1 Patient is steady with eyes open but becomes unsteady when eyes are closed = positive Romberg's sign indicating presence of sensory ataxia.
2 Patient is equally unsteady both with eyes opened and closed = cerebellar ataxia.

Titubations (to and fro or rotatory head tremors):
1 Cerebellar dysfunction.
2 Part of essential tremors.

Chorea/choreiform movements:
1 Sydenham's chorea (rheumatic fever).
2 Huntington's chorea.
3 Wilson's disease.
4 Cerebellar degeneration.
5 Pregnancy (chorea gravidarum).
6 Polycythaemia rubra vera.
7 SLE.
8 Thyrotoxicosis.
9 Drug-induced (neuroleptics [dopamine antagonists]; phenytoin; OCPs).

Myoclonus:
1 Physiologic when falling asleep.
2 Epilepsy.
3 Organ failure (hepatic; renal).

Hemiballismus:
1 Lesion is in the contralateral subthalamic nucleus.

Gait abnormalities:

1 Bizarre gait with exaggerated delay on affected limb:
   a Functional.
2 Spastic gait (feet not lifted off the ground completely so that toes remain in contact with the ground at all times):
   a UMN paraplegia.
   b Hemiplegia (also called hemiplegic gait).
3 Stiff leg swung in an arc:
   a Contralateral pyramidal tract lesion (in cerebral hemisphere, internal capsule, brainstem or spinal cord).
4 Shuffling gait (steps are smaller than normal):
   a Parkinsonism.
5 Festinant gait (patient bends forward and takes rapid small steps in an attempt to maintain an upright posture):
   a Parkinsonism.
6 High-stepping gait:
   a Bilateral foot-drop (as can occur in polyneuropathy cases).
7 Wide-based gait:
   a Cerebellar disease (tumour, ischaemia, etc).
   b Drug effect (wide-based gait, nystagmus, past-pointing and h/o alcohol/drug intake).
8 Drunken gait (broad-based gait with patient reeling towards the side of lesion):
   a Cerebellar lesion.
9 Bilateral stamping, high-stepping gait:
   a Dorsal column lesion.
   b Peripheral neuropathy (d/t vitamin B_{12} deficiency, etc).
10 Unilateral stamping, high-stepping gait:
   a Lateral popliteal nerve palsy.
11 Scissors or wading-through-mud gait:
   a Bilateral UMN lesion (usually in the spinal cord).
12 Waddling gait (body sways from side to side while walking; hip tilts down when the leg is lifted):
   a Pelvic girdle and proximal muscle weakness (d/t hereditary muscular dystrophy).
   b Congenital dislocation of the hip joints.
13 Hobbling with minimal time spent on the affected limb:
   a Bone, joint or muscle pathology.

Proximal myopathy (difficulty in rising from chair or squatting position):

1 Muscle pathology (diabetic amyotrophy; dermatomyositis; polymyositis; hereditary dystrophy [positive family history]; carcinomatous neuromyopathy).
2 Endocrinopathy (thyrotoxicosis; Cushing's syndrome).

3 Osteomalacia.

Apraxia (in the absence of any motor or sensory deficit, patient unable to perform common actions like combing the hair, buttoning the shirt or drawing a square on the paper):
  1 Bilateral apraxia:
     a Lesion is the dominant parietal lobe.
  2 Unilateral apraxia involving non-dominant limb only:
     a Lesion is the non-dominant parietal lobe.

Hemisection of the spinal cord (Brown–Séquard's syndrome):
  1 Ipsilateral UMN weakness and loss of position and vibration senses.
  2 Contralateral loss of pain and temperature senses.

Barber's chair sign (touch the chest with the chin rapidly → electric shock like sensations down the arm/spine/legs):
  1 Lesion is in the midcervical region; d/t cervical spondylosis, syringomyelia, multiple sclerosis or B_{12} deficiency.

Astereognosis:
  1 Lesion is in the sensory cortex.

Features of sensory cortex damage:
Loss of:
  1 Sense of localisation.
  2 Two-point discrimination.
  3 Stereognosis.
  4 Graphaesthesia.

Presence of:
  1 Perceptual rivalry.

Dementia:
CNS diseases:
  1 Alzheimer's disease.
  2 Lewy-body dementia.
  3 Multi-infarct dementia.
  4 Huntington's disease.
  5 Parkinsonism.
  6 Pick's disease.
  7 Creutzfeld–Jakob's disease (CJD).
  8 Acute or chronic head injury.
  9 SOL.
  10 Normal-pressure hydrocephalus.

Thyroid disease:
1 Hypothyroidism.

Nutritional/malabsorption:
1 Chronic alcoholism/chronic substance abuse.
2 Severe niacin/vitamin B_{12}/folic acid deficiency.

Liver disease:
1 Wilson's disease.

Potentially treatable causes of dementia:
1 CNS disease:
   a Normal-pressure hydrocephalus.
2 Thyroid disease:
   a Hypothyroidism.
3 Nutritional/malabsorption:
   a Niacin/vitamin B_{12}/folic acid deficiency.
4 Liver disease:
   a Wilson's disease.

Leg pain on walking – intermittent claudication:
1 Peripheral arterial disease (associated impotence = Leriche's syndrome) – cold toes d/t poor perfusion, and abnormal pulses.
2 Spinal claudication – no cold toes, normal pulses.

Leg pain on standing; relieved by lying down:
1 Peripheral venous disease/varicose veins.
2 Slipped disc.

Common peroneal nerve palsy (L4, L5, S1, S2):
1 Fracture neck of fibula.
2 Weight loss.
3 Diabetes mellitus.
4 PAN.
5 Leprosy.

Fatigue (tired all the time):
Generally a poor lead, but consider the following:
1 Depression.
2 Chronic fatigue syndrome.
3 Diabetes mellitus.
4 Sleep problem (long working hours → little sleep; insomnia d/t any reason; sleep-apnoea syndrome).
5 Parasomnias (restless legs; cataplexy; narcolepsy; daytime somnolence).

6 Postviral fatigue (especially glandular fever).

7 Drug-induced (sedatives; antiepileptics).

Headache:

1 Tension headache.

2 Referred headache (from ophthalmic,[8] ENT[9] or dental problems[10]).

3 Vascular headache (fever; migraine; cluster headache;[11] high blood pressure;[12] temporal arteritis; hypercapnia d/t type-II respiratory failure → cerebral vasodilatation → headache).

4 SOL (like haematoma; abscess; cyst; tumour; AVM).

5 Meningitis/encephalitis/meningoencephalitis/intracerebral haemorrhage /SAH.

6 Cranial neuralgias:

   a Trigeminal neuralgia:

     i Old patient – idiopathic (commonest cause).

     ii Young patient – multiple sclerosis.

     iii Postherpetic.

     iv Nerve compression (d/t a redundant/tortuous blood vessel in the posterior cranial fossa – rare).

   b Glossopharyngeal neuralgia.

7 Drug side effect: e.g. nitrates.

Epilepsy:

1 Idiopathic (usually starts in childhood).

2 Head injury.

3 SOL (like haematoma; abscess; cyst; tumour; AVM).

4 Cerebrovascular accident.

5 Infection (meningitis; encephalitis; cerebral malaria; tetanus; febrile fits in children;[13] scar epilepsy).

6 Deranged blood chemistry ($\downarrow$ glucose; $\downarrow$ Ca^{2+}; $\downarrow$ Mg^{2+}; $\downarrow$ Na^{+}; $\uparrow$ K^{+}).

7 Organ failure (renal, hepatic, respiratory failure).

8 Sudden severe hypotension (d/t cardiac arrest, etc) → anoxic brain damage.

9 Alcohol withdrawal.

10 Functional (pseudo-fits): always occurring in front of audience; eyes closed during episode.

---

8   Refractive error (myopia; presbyopia); iritis; glaucoma.

9   Sinusitis (frontal; ethmoidal; maxillary); otitis externa/media/mastoiditis.

10 Dental abscesses, etc.

11 Also called migrainous neuralgia.

12 It includes both systemic HTN and benign intracranial HTN (also called pseudotumour cerebri).

13 Febrile fits occur in children. These should not be taken as indicative of epilepsy unless recurrent.

Pregnant women presenting with epilepsy:
1 Eclampsia.
2 HELLP syndrome (haemolysis + ↑ LFTs + ↓ platelets).
3 TTP.[14]
4 CNS pathology (SOL; cerebral haemorrhage; cerebral vein thrombosis secondary to hyperviscosity).

Classification of convulsions (seizures):
1 Partial or focal seizures:
 a Simple partial seizures.
 b Complex partial seizures.
2 Generalised seizures:
 a Primary generalised seizures.
 b Secondary generalised seizures (d/t SOL; do CT/MRI scan).

Features of partial seizures:
1 Contraction of a part of the body, e.g. hand or face; it may spread to the other parts – called Jacksonian march.
2 Visual or auditory hallucinations may be present.
3 No alteration of consciousness – called 'simple' partial seizures; conscious level altered – called 'complex' partial seizures.

Features of secondary generalised seizures:
In the following order:
1 Aura: unusual smell; illusion of objects growing smaller (micropsia) or larger (macropsia); visual hallucinations; sudden intense emotional feeling.
2 Focal features: twitching of an extremity; aphasia.
3 Generalised seizures.
4 Todd's paralysis (postictal focal neurological deficit).

Classification of epilepsy (continuing tendency to have seizures):
1 Partial or focal epilepsy:
 a Temporal lobe epilepsy ('psychomotor' epilepsy).
 b Jacksonian epilepsy.
2 Generalised epilepsy:
 a Tonic–clonic epilepsy.
 b Tonic epilepsy.
 c Absence seizures (petit mal epilepsy).

---

14 TTP = MAHA + thrombocytopenia + fever + renal/CNS involvement. Not all patients have this classic pentad. Usually MAHA and thrombocytopenia are required to make the diagnosis.

Investigations for epilepsy:

1 EEG: should be done in every patient; always abnormal during attack; normal between attacks.
2 Radiological investigations:[15] X-ray skull; CT/MRI scan; isotope brain scan; cerebral angiography.

Cerebellar signs:

1 Eye: nystagmus.
2 Speech: dysarthria (scanning speech).
3 Upper limb: intention tremors; incoordination (past-pointing present – checked by finger–nose and shin–heel tests); dysdiadochokinesia; rebound phenomenon.
4 Lower limb: hypotonia; pendular knee jerk; shin–heel test.
5 Romberg's test: cerebellar ataxia.
6 Gait: ataxia (reeling and broad-based gait – patient tends to fall towards the side of lesion).

GCS:

Eye opening (E):	
Spontaneous	4
To speech	3
To pain	2
Nil	1
Verbal response (V):	
Oriented	5
Confused conversation	4
Inappropriate words	3
Incomprehensible sounds	2
Nil	1
Motor response (M):	
Obeys	6
Localises	5
Withdraws	4
Flexor response	3
Extensor response	2
Nil	1

---

15 Done if patient is not a child and fits have started for the first time after childhood; history suggests partial, or secondary generalised seizures; papilloedema is found on clinical examination; past h/o persistent headache or vomiting is present.

Interpretation: EMV minimum = 3; maximum = 15

GCS = 15: probably no brain damage currently.

GCS = 13–15: minor brain damage.

GCS = 9–12: moderate brain damage.

GCS = 3–8: severe brain damage/deep coma.

GCS = 3: very severe brain damage/death.

Edinburgh coma scale:
- Grade-I: confused but responds to verbal commands.
- Grade-II: responds to minimal painful stimuli only.
- Grade-II: responds to maximal painful stimuli only.
- Grade-IV: no response.

Dizziness:
1 Psychogenic (panic attack).
2 CNS disease (epilepsy).
3 Carotid sinus hypersensitivity.
4 Anaemia.
5 Postural hypotension.
6 Hypoxia.
7 Drugs (sedatives; hypotensives; alcohol).

Tremors:
Tremors at rest:
1 Parkinsonism.

Intention tremors:
1 Cerebellar disease.

Action tremors:
1 Anxiety.
2 Thyrotoxicosis.
3 Flapping tremors.
4 Senile tremors.
5 Essential familial tremors.
6 Alcohol withdrawal.
7 Sympathomimetic drugs (e.g. amphetamines).

Fine tremors of the outstretched hand:
1 Anxiety.
2 Thyrotoxicosis.
3 Flapping tremors.
4 Senile tremors.
5 Essential familial tremors.

6 Alcohol withdrawal.

7 Sympathomimetic drugs.

Coarse tremors of the hand:

1 Organ failure (hepatic; pulmonary [d/t CO_2 retention]).

2 Parkinsonism.

3 Cerebellar disease.

4 Essential familial tremors.

Parkinsonism:

1 Parkinson's disease.

2 Drug-induced (metoclopramide; chlorpromazine; prochlorperazine; haloperidol).

3 Dementia (Alzheimer's dementia; Lewy-body dementia; dementia pugilistica[16]).

4 Post encephalitis.

5 Normal-pressure hydrocephalus.

6 Multisystem atrophy.

Abnormal posture of arms and hand at rest:

1 Flexion at elbow and wrist joints + UMN-type weakness of the upper limb and facial muscles:

   a Lesion of contralateral precentral gyrus, internal capsule or lower pyramidal tract.

2 Claw hand:

   a T1 anterior root lesion (claw hand + wasting of all small muscles of the hand + loss of sensation along ulnar border of the forearm and ulnar 1.5 fingers).

   b Ulnar nerve lesion – below elbow (claw hand + wasting of hypothenar eminence + dorsal guttering esp. first + weakness of finger abduction and adduction + loss of sensation along ulnar 1.5 fingers).

3 Wrist-drop and inability to grip + loss of sensation over 1st dorsal inter-osseous muscle.

   a Radial nerve (C7 anterior root) lesion.

Muscle wasting:

1 Adjacent bone or joint disease.

2 LMN type lesion.

3 Primary muscle pathology.

Wasting of the small muscles of the hand:

1 T1 lesion (anterior horn cell or root lesion):

---

16 Caused by chronic head injury, e.g. from boxing.

a Syringomyelia.
b Cervical rib.
c Cervical spondylosis[17] (compressing nerve root).
d Tumour compressing T1 root/Pancoast's tumour.
e Brachial plexus lesion.
f MND.
2 Ulnar nerve paralysis (at elbow or wrist).
3 Median nerve paralysis (usually d/t carpal tunnel syndrome).
4 Polyneuropathy.
5 Any prolonged systemic illness.

Wasting of arm and shoulder:
1 MND (amyotrophic lateral sclerosis with anterior horn cell degeneration; progressive muscle atrophy).
2 Primary muscle pathology.

Abnormal arm tone:
1 ↓ tone:
  a Cerebellar pathology.
  b Primary muscle pathology.
2 ↑ tone:
  a UMN lesion.
  b Parkinson's disease.

Incoordination on rapid wrist rotation or hand tapping:
1 ↑ tone in the upper limb:
  a UMN-type paresis.
2 ↓ tone in the upper limb:
  a LMN-type paresis.
  b Ipsilateral cerebellar lesion (↓ tone + diminished reflexes + past-pointing).
3 Loss of proprioception:
  a Dorsal column lesion.

Weakness of shoulder/arm without pain:
1 C4–5 root lesion: (weakness of abduction at the shoulder – not at elbow or wrist).
2 C5–6 root lesion (Erb's palsy): weakness of flexion at shoulder and elbow but not at wrist; arm externally rotated and adducted behind back in 'porter's tip' position; usually in neonates with h/o birth trauma.
3 C7 root lesion: wrist-drop or weakness of extension at the wrist (→ weak grip) and elbow.

---

17 Cervical spondylosis = cervical disc degeneration ± herniation.

4 Radial nerve lesion: wrist-drop or weakness of extension at the wrist ($\rightarrow$ weak grip) but not at the elbow.

5 C8-T1 root lesion (Klumpke's palsy): arm held in adduction, paralysis/ paresis of the small muscles of the hand, loss of sensation over ulnar border of the hand. Usually in neonates with h/o birth trauma.

Weakness of hip flexion alone:
1 L1–2 root lesion or femoral nerve lesion.

Weakness of hip adduction alone:
1 L2–3 root lesion or obturator nerve lesion.

Weakness of knee extension alone:
1 L3–4 root lesion or femoral nerve lesion.

Weakness of knee flexion alone:
1 L5–S1 root lesion or common peroneal nerve lesion.

Weakness of foot dorsiflexion and ankle inversion:
1 L4–5 root lesion or tibial nerve lesion.

Foot-drop with weakness of foot dorsiflexion and ankle eversion (and loss of sensation along the lateral aspect of the leg:
1 Lateral popliteal nerve palsy (usually traumatic).

Weakness of toe flexion alone:
1 S1–2 root lesion or sciatic nerve lesion.

Bilateral weakness of all foot movements:
1 GB syndrome.
2 Lead poisoning.
3 Porphyria.
4 Charcot–Marie–Tooth's disease.

Disturbed sensation in the upper limb:
1 Higher cortical sensations lost (diminished 2-point discrimination, astereognosis and graphaesthesia):
   a Contralateral precentral gyrus lesion.
2 Loss of touch and pinprick sensation in the hand and to variable extent proximally:
   a Peripheral neuropathy.
3 Loss of pinprick and temperature sensation:
   a Spinothalamic tract lesion (d/t syringomyelia). Touch may be normal or disturbed; normal position and vibration sensation in the hand.

4 Loss of sensation in a dermatome:
   a Cervical or thoracic nerve root lesion.
5 Localised loss of sensation (in arm, forearm, radial 3.5 or ulnar 1.5 fingers):
   a Peripheral nerve lesion.

Loss of sensation along the lateral aspect of upper arm:
1 C5 posterior root lesion.

Loss of sensation along the inner aspect of upper arm and breast:
1 T2 posterior root lesion.

Loss of sensation along the lateral forearm and thumb:
1 C6 posterior root lesion.

Loss of sensation along the ulnar border of the forearm:
1 T1 posterior root lesion.

Loss of sensation along the palmar aspect of radial 3.5 fingers:
1 Medial nerve lesion.

Loss of sensation along the dorsal aspect of radial 3.5 fingers:
1 Radial nerve lesion.

Loss of sensation of the middle finger alone:
1 C7 posterior root lesion.

Loss of sensation along the ulnar 1.5 fingers (both dorsal and ventral aspects) and the ulnar border of the wrist:
1 C8 posterior root lesion.

Loss of sensation along ulnar 1.5 fingers (both dorsal and ventral aspects) but not the ulnar border of the wrist:
1 Ulnar nerve lesion.

Medial nerve lesion:
1 Carpal tunnel syndrome/local nerve trauma.
2 Rheumatoid arthritis.
3 Endocrinopathy (acromegaly; hypothyroidism),
4 OCPs.
5 Pregnancy.

Ulnar nerve lesion:
1 At wrist (deep palmar branch affected):
   a Trauma.

2 At elbow (ulnar groove):
  a Trauma.
  b Osteoarthritis.

Radial nerve lesion:

1 'Saturday night' palsy (arm left hanging over chair).

C7 posterior root lesion:

1 Cervical spondylosis (compression by osteophytes).

C8 posterior root lesion:

1 Cervical spondylosis (compression by osteophytes).

Disturbed sensation in the lower limb:

1 Higher cortical sensations lost (graphaesthesia):
  a Contralateral precentral gyrus lesion.
2 Loss of touch and pinprick sensation in the foot and to variable extent proximally:
  a Peripheral neuropathy.
3 Loss of pinprick and temperature sensation:
  a Spinothalamic tract lesion (d/t contralateral hemisection of the spinal cord). Touch may be normal or disturbed; normal position and vibration sensation in the hand.
4 Loss of position and vibration sensation in the foot (pinprick and temperature intact):
  a Dorsal column lesion.
5 Loss of sensation in the inguinal region:
  a L1 posterior root lesion.
6 Loss of sensation in the anterior thigh:
  a L2–3 posterior root lesion.
7 Loss of sensation in the anterior shin:
  a L4–5 posterior root lesion.
8 Loss of sensation along the lateral border of the foot:
  a S1 posterior root lesion.

Dissociated anaesthesia (loss of pain and temperature sensation; preservation of touch):

1 Syringomyelia*.
2 Syringobulbia* (dilatation of the central canal of brainstem).
3 Tumours of the central canal of the spinal cord*.

* T_1 compression → wasting of the small muscles of the hand.

Carpal tunnel syndrome:

1 Tendon disease (localised tenosynovitis).
2 Joint disease (rheumatoid arthritis).
3 Endocrine disease (myxoedema; acromegaly).
4 Pregnancy.
5 OCPs.
6 Amyloidosis.

Coma – (GCS score ≤8):
1 CNS disease (infection; CVA; SOL; epilepsy [post epileptic fit; status epilepticus]; head injury).
2 Diabetic coma (DKA; hyperosmolar non-ketotic coma; lactic acidosis; hypoglycaemic coma).
3 Organ failure (renal, hepatic, respiratory failure).
4 Electrolytes disturbances ($\downarrow$ Na$^+$; $\uparrow$ Na$^+$).
5 Hyperpyrexia (rectal temperature ≥41°C />106°F).
6 Septicaemia.
7 Drug overdose/poisoning – common poisons:
  a Antidepressants.
  b Benzodiazepines.
  c Barbiturates.
  d Corrosives.
  e Morphine and its derivatives.
  f Pesticides.
  g PCM/dextropropoxyphene.
  h Salicylates.

Last two are common in the west.

Low CSF glucose (with normal plasma glucose):
1 Meningeal irritation:
  a Meningitis (bacterial/tuberculous).
  b Meningeal carcinomatosis.
  c Subarachnoid haemorrhage.

High CSF proteins:
1 Meningeal irritation:
  a Meningitis (bacterial/tuberculous/fungal).
  b Meningeal carcinomatosis.
  c Subarachnoid haemorrhage.
2 Guillain–Barré's syndrome.
3 Transverse myelitis.
4 Spinal block (secondary to tumour).
5 Acoustic neuroma.

Markedly raised (2–6 g/L) CSF proteins:

1 GB syndrome.
2 Spinal block (secondary to tumour).
3 Tuberculous/fungal meningitis.

High CSF proteins with normal CSF cell count:

1 GB syndrome.
2 Malignancy (spinal cord tumour → spinal block [called Froin's syndrome]; acoustic neuroma).
3 Encephalopathy (lead encephalopathy; subacute sclerosing panencephalopathy).

Lymphocytosis and ↑ CSF proteins:

1 Infection: viral/tuberculous/partially treated bacterial/cryptococcal meningitis; listeria; leptospirosis; Lyme disease; brucellosis; HIV; toxoplasmosis; neurosyphilis; cerebral abscess.
2 Non-infective:
   a Stroke.
   b Malignancy (cerebral lymphoma/leukaemia/metastases).
   c Granulomatous disease (sarcoidosis).
   d CT disorder (SLE).
   e Behçet's syndrome.
   f Multiple sclerosis.

↑ Lymphocytes in the CSF:

1 Same as above.

↑ CSF Pressure:

1 SOL.
2 Hydrocephalus.
3 Dural sinus thrombosis.
4 Benign intracranial hypertension.

Dural sinus thrombosis:

1 Infection of the face, ears or sinuses.
2 OCPs/pregnancy.
3 Behçet's syndrome.
4 Hereditary thrombophilic states.
5 Hyperviscosity states.

Transient neurological deficit:

1 Thromboembolic phenomenon (embolus from carotid artery stenosis or vasculitic process; heart secondary to AF/valvular lesion).
2 SOL (haematoma; abscess; tumour; cyst; aneurysm; AVM).

3 Other CNS pathologies (multiple sclerosis; migraine; Todd's paralysis following epileptic fit).
4 Transient hypotension (d/t MI or arrhythmia).
5 Metabolic cause (hypoglycaemic episode; hyponatraemia).
6 Psychological.

Hemiplegia: nature of lesion:
1 CVA/stroke:
   a Haemorrhagic: SAH (primary/secondary); intracerebral haemorrhage.
   b Infarctive: thrombosis; embolism.
2 SOL (haematoma; abscess; cysts; tumour; AVM).

CVA/stroke:
Infarction/ischaemic stroke:
1 Cerebral thrombosis.
2 Cerebral embolism.

Haemorrhage:
1 Intracerebral haemorrhage.
2 Subarachnoid haemorrhage.

Risk factors for CVA/stroke:
1 HTN.
2 DM.
3 Smoking.
4 Hyperlipidaemia.
5 Positive family history.

Uncrossed hemiplegia[18] – site of lesion:
1 Motor cortex (precentral gyrus of frontal lobe):
   a Monoplegia; Jacksonian fits may occur.
2 Corona radiata:
   a Hemiparesis (one limb involved more than the other).
3 Internal capsule:
   a Complete hemiplegia; cortical sensory loss and hemianopia may occur.

Crossed hemiplegia[19] – site of lesion:
1 Midbrain:

---

18 Hemiplegia and CN involvement are on the same side.

19 Hemiplegia and CN involvement are on the opposite sides. Lesion is in the brainstem on the side of CN involvement.

a 3rd or 4th cranial nerves involved; bilaterally dilated (>6 mm) and fixed pupils may be present (it signifies severe midbrain damage).
2 Pons:
   a One or more of 5th, 6th, 7th or 8th nerves involved; pinpoint (<1 mm) and reacting pupils; hyperpyrexia may occur.
3 Medulla oblongata:
   a One or more of 9th, 10th, 11th or 12th nerves involved.

Cerebral embolism – sources:
1 Atheroma of the extra- or intracranial vessels (carotid bruit; weak carotid pulses).
2 Heart:
   a Arrhythmias (AF, etc).
   b Recent MI.
   c Infective endocarditis.
   d Valvular heart disease (mitral or aortic).
   e Prosthetic valve.

Intracerebral haemorrhage:
1 HTN.
2 Aneurysm/AVM.
3 Vasculitis
4 Bleeding disorder.

Subarachnoid haemorrhage (SAH):
1 Primary:
   a Trauma.
   b HTN.
   c Berry aneurysm/aneurysm of the posterior communicating artery/ AVM.
   d Vasculitis.
   e Bleeding disorder.
   f Cocaine/amphetamine abuse.
2 Secondary:
   a Extension of intracerebral haemorrhage into the subarachnoid space.

SAH: complications:
1 Neurological deficit.
2 Rebleed (30%).
3 Hydrocephalus.
4 SIADH.

Berry aneurysm – associations:
1 Renal pathology (ADPKD; renal artery stenosis).

2 Vasculitis (PAN).

3 Ehlers–Danlos' syndrome.

Hemiparesis:

1 Middle cerebral artery infarction:
  a Upper branch occluded (Broca's area involved → expressive dysphasia + contralateral lower face and arm weakness).
  b Perforating branch occluded (→ hemiparesis alone with subsequent spasticity, or hemianaesthesia alone, or receptive dysphasia alone).
  c Total occlusion – usually embolic (→ contralateral flaccid hemiplegia [with little subsequent spasticity] + hemianaesthesia + deviation of head towards the side of lesion + aphasia and homonymous hemianopia if dominant hemisphere is affected or 'neglect' if non-dominant hemisphere is affected).

2 Posterior cerebral artery infarction:
  a Mild contralateral hemiparesis, ataxia, involuntary movements and sensory loss, ipsilateral 3rd nerve palsy, contralateral homonymous hemianopia or upper quadrantanopia, dyslexia and memory loss.

3 Anterior cerebral artery infarction:
  a Weakness and rigidity of the contralateral leg, perseveration, urinary incontinence, grasp reflex in opposite hand and dysphasia if the lesion is in the dominant hemisphere.

Features of various arterial aneurysms:

1 Internal carotid artery:
  a Within cavernous sinus:
    i 3rd, 4th or 6th nerve palsy.
    ii Pain and paraesthesias in the distribution of ophthalmic division of 5th nerve.
    iii Caroticocavernous fistula.
  b Supraclinoid part:
    i Compression of optic nerve, optic chiasma or optic tract leading to visual field defects.
    ii 3rd nerve palsy.

2 Middle cerebral artery:
  a Progressive hemiparesis.
  b Focal epilepsy.

3 Anterior cerebral and anterior communicating arteries:
  a Compression of optic chiasma → bitemporal hemianopia.

4 Posterior communicating artery:
  a Isolated 3rd nerve palsy.

5 Posterior cerebral artery:
  a Isolated 3rd nerve palsy + contralateral hemiplegia.

Hemiplegia in a comatose patient:
1 Up-going plantar on one side – highly suggestive.
2 Bilaterally up-going plantars – no localising value.

Cortical sensory functions:[20]
1 Tactile localisation.
2 Two-point discrimination.
3 Stereognosis.[21]

Prefrontal lobe[22] – localising signs:
1 Personality changes (disinhibited; abnormal affective reaction; indifferent; lack of concentration; difficulty with planning and initiative; lack of concern over consequences of an action; perseveration[23]).
2 Anosmia.
3 Micturition disturbances.
4 Primitive reflexes positive (e.g. grasp reflex positive).

Precentral gyrus[24] – localising signs:
1 Contralateral hemiparesis/hemiplegia.
2 Jacksonian fits.
3 Motor dysphasia (if dominant hemisphere involved).

Parietal lobe – localising signs:
Features common to both hemispheres:
1 Homonymous lower quadrantanopia.
2 Apraxia.[25]
3 Loss of cortical sensory functions.

Additional features of dominant hemisphere:
1 Gerstmann's syndrome.[26]
2 Alexia (inability to read).
3 Tactile agnosia (bimanual astereognosis).
4 Sensory dysphasia.

---

20 If absent, it signifies damage to the sensory cortex (postcentral gyrus).
21 Inability to identify common objects by palpation with one hand (opposite: astereognosis).
22 Area anterior to the motor area involved.
23 Constant repetition of meaningless words or phrases.
24 Motor area involved.
25 Inability to perform a learned act in the absence of any motor deficit or joint disease.
26 Inability to distinguish b/w right and left; finger agnosia; agraphia; acalculia.

Additional features of non-dominant hemisphere:
1 Spatial disorientation (unable to find way around).
2 Sensory inattention (perceptual rivalry).[27]
3 Anosognosia (unaware of paralysis).
4 Autotopagnosia (ignores paralysed side).

Temporal lobe – localising signs:
1 Homonymous upper quadrantanopia of the opposite side.
2 Cortical deafness (when auditory cortex is involved bilaterally).
3 Auditory or olfactory hallucinations.
4 Auditory or visual illusions.
5 Déjà vu phenomenon.
6 Automatism.

Occipital lobe – localising signs:
1 Homonymous hemianopia of the opposite side.
2 Visual hallucinations.

Normal-pressure hydrocephalus:
1 Primary.
2 Secondary:
   a Head injury.
   b Meningitis.
   c SAH.

Benign intracranial hypertension:
1 Drug-induced:
   a OCPs.
   b Steroids.
   c Antibiotics (tetracycline; nalidixic acid; nitrofurantoin).
   d Vitamin A.

Up-going plantars:
1 UMN lesion.
2 Deep coma.
3 Post epileptic fit.
4 Hypoglycaemia.
5 1st year of life (physiological).

Up-going plantars with absent ankle jerk:
1 Subacute combined degeneration of the spinal cord.

---

27 When both sides (e.g. both legs) are touched separately, patient can recognise them, but when they are touched simultaneously, side opposite to the affected parietal lobe is ignored.

2 Tabes dorsalis (neurosyphilis).
3 Friedreich's ataxia.

Upper motor neuron (UMN) type paraplegia – common causes:
1 Spinal cord compression.
2 Subacute combined degeneration of the spinal cord.
3 Transverse myelitis.
4 Multiple sclerosis affecting the spinal cord.
5 Motor neuron disease (amyotrophic lateral sclerosis).
6 Friedreich's ataxia.

Upper motor neuron (UMN) type paraplegia – uncommon causes:
1 Hereditary spastic paraplegia (HSP).
2 Tabes dorsalis (neurosyphilis).
3 Syringomyelia.
4 Spinal cord infarction.
5 Intracranial lesions (thrombosis of sagittal sinus; parasagittal meningioma).

Upper motor neuron (UMN) type paraplegia of sudden onset:
1 Spinal cord compression (must be excluded).
2 Spinal cord infarction.
3 Transverse myelitis.

Spinal cord compression:
Extradural:
1 Trauma (vertebral fracture; disc herniation).
2 Infection (TB; abscess) or malignancy of the spinal column (myeloma; metastases).

Extramedullary:
1 Meningioma.
2 AVM.

Intramedullary:
1 Tumour of the spinal cord.

Lower motor neuron (LMN) type paraplegia:
1 Guillain–Barré's syndrome (postinfective polyneuritis).
2 Compression of the cauda equina.
3 Peripheral neuropathy/poliomyelitis.
4 Myopathy (thyrotoxicosis; Cushing's syndrome; dermatomyositis/polymyositis; muscular dystrophy; progressive muscular atrophy; osteomalacia).

5 Hypo-[28]/normo-/hyperkalaemic periodic paralysis.

6 Hysterical.

Paraplegia with abnormal CSF findings:
UMN paraplegia:
1 Inflammatory lesions (abscess; TB):
    a ↑ cell number.
2 Transverse myelitis:
    a ↑ CSF proteins + up to 50 lymphocytes/μL.
3 Malignancy:
    a Malignant cells seen.
4 Multiple sclerosis:
    a ↑ oligoclonal IgG.
5 Froin's syndrome (spinal cord blockage → blockage of CSF flow):
    a Yellow-coloured CSF (xanthochromia) + ↑ CSF proteins (markedly increased) + Queckenstedt's test positive.[29]

LMN paraplegia:
1 GB syndrome:
    a ↑ proteins; cell count remains within the normal limit. This is called protein–cell dissociation.

Quadriplegia:
1 Bilateral stroke.
2 LMN paraplegia (d/t any cause) can ascend and cause quadriplegia.
3 UMN paraplegia (→ quadriplegia):
    a Compression of the cervical cord in the cervical region.
    b Syringomyelia.
    c Transverse myelitis.
    d Amyotrophic lateral sclerosis.

Respiratory paralysis:
1 Transection/compression of upper cervical spinal cord.
2 Transverse myelitis.
3 GB syndrome.
4 Myasthenia gravis.
5 Botulism.

---

28 Thyrotoxic hypokalaemic periodic paralysis: thyrotoxicosis (↑ T4, ↑ T3 and undetectable TSH) + h/o heavy exertion ↑ CPK and ↓ K⁺ → muscle weakness.

29 Measure CSF pressure during LP. Then press the jugular vein in the neck. It should cause a sudden rise in the CSF pressure; if not, it suggests a blockage in the spinal canal. If so, the Queckenstedt's test is positive.

6 In most patients with motor neuron disease and muscular dystrophies (as part of the terminal illness).
7 K⁺-related periodic paralysis.
8 Snake bite.

Anterior cord/spinal syndrome (anterior spinal artery obstructed):
1 Flaccid/spastic paraparesis.
2 Loss of pain and temperature sensation bilaterally.
3 Dorsal columns intact.

Brown–Séquard's syndrome (lateral hemisection of the cord):
1 Ipsilateral UMN weakness below the lesion.
2 Ipsilateral loss of position and vibration sensation.
3 Contralateral loss of pain and temperature sensation.

Autonomic neuropathy:
1 Diabetes mellitus.
2 Organ failure (hepatic; renal).
3 Amyloidosis.
4 GB syndrome.
5 Multiple nervous system atrophies (e.g. Shy–Drager's syndrome).

Polyneuropathy:
1 Idiopathic.
2 Metabolic (diabetes mellitus; uraemia; amyloidosis; porphyria).
3 Vitamin deficiency (B_1, B_6, B_{12}).
4 Drugs (INH; nitrofurantoin; vincristine; heavy metals).
5 Inflammation (CT disorders); infection (botulism; diphtheria; leprosy; tetanus); malignancy; GB syndrome.
6 Compressive neuropathy (e.g. carpal tunnel syndrome).
7 Hereditary:
  a Friedreich's ataxia.
  b Charcot–Marie–Tooth's disease (peroneal muscular atrophy).
  c Dejerine–Sottas' disease (hypertrophic interstitial neuritis).

Polyneuropathy – primarily sensory:
1 Diabetes mellitus.
2 Uraemia.
3 Amyloidosis.
4 Vitamin B_{12} deficiency.
5 Leprosy.

Polyneuropathy – primarily motor:
1 Diphtheria.

2 GB syndrome.

3 Porphyria.

4 Lead intoxication.

Thickened peripheral nerves:

1 HSMN[30] type III (also called Dejerine–Sottas' disease).

2 Acromegaly.

3 Neurofibromatosis.

4 Infection (tuberculoid leprosy; HIV).

Simultaneous CVS and CNS disease – infections:

1 TB.

2 Rheumatic fever/infective endocarditis.

3 Lyme disease.

4 Syphilis.

Simultaneous CVS and CNS disease – multisystem conditions:

1 GB syndrome

2 CT disorders (SLE; RA).

3 Sarcoidosis.

4 Acute intermittent porphyria.

5 Vasculitides.

Simultaneous CVS and CNS disease – hereditary neuropathies:

1 Friedreich's ataxia.

2 Duchenne's muscular dystrophy.

3 Dystrophia myotonica.

Simultaneous CVS and CNS disease – neuroectodermal syndromes:

1 Neurofibromatosis.

2 Tuberous sclerosis.

Simultaneous CVS and CNS disease – drugs/toxins:

1 TCAs.

2 Lithium.

3 Recreational agents (amphetamines; alcohol).

---

30 Hereditary sensorimotor neuropathy.

7 Haematology

Lymphadenopathy:
1 Disease in the 'drainage area' (infection or malignancy).
2 Granulomatous disease (TB; sarcoidosis).
3 Infection (infectious mononucleosis; viral hepatitis; HIV).
4 Malignancy (lymphoma; leukaemia).

Hilar lymphadenopathy:
1 Granulomatous disease (primary TB; sarcoidosis).
2 Malignancy (ca. lung; metastases; Hodgkin's or non-Hodgkin's lymphoma).

Groin lymphadenopathy:
1 Infection somewhere in the lower limb or pelvis (usually d/t a past infection with persistent lymphadenopathy).

Generalised lymphadenopathy:
1 Granulomatous disease (sarcoidosis).
2 Infection (infectious mononucleosis; HIV).
3 Malignancy (lymphoma; leukaemia).
4 Drugs (phenytoin; retroviral therapy).

Staging of Hodgkin's lymphoma:
Four stages:
1 Stage-I: involvement of a single lymph node region or extralymphatic site.
2 Stage-II: involvement of ≥2 lymph node regions or extralymphatic sites on one side of the diaphragm.
3 Stage-III: involvement of lymph node regions or extralymphatic sites on both sides of the diaphragm, or splenic involvement.
4 Stage-IV: diffuse involvement of liver or bone marrow.
   a symptoms absent.
   b one or more of the symptoms are present (unexplained weight loss of >10% of the body weight; unexplained fever of >38°C/100.4°F; night sweats).

Histological classification of Hodgkin's lymphoma:
Four subtypes:
1 Lymphocyte predominant.
2 Lymphocyte-depleted.

3 Mixed cellularity.

4 Nodular sclerosing.

Complications of lymphoma:

1 Effects of exogenous compression (dysphagia; SVC/IVC obstruction; intestinal obstruction).

2 Respiratory distress.

3 Ascites.

4 Paraplegia.

5 Bone pains.

Normocytic anaemia:

1 Acute blood loss.

2 Anaemia of pregnancy.

3 Anaemia of chronic disease (CRF; chronic inflammation, e.g. CT disorders;[1] chronic infections, e.g. TB; malignancy – without infiltrating bone marrow; hypogonadism).

4 Bone marrow suppression[2] (idiopathic; viral infection – HBV; malignancy – leukaemia;[3] iatrogenic: drugs – chloramphenicol, cytotoxics, e.g. hydroxycarbamide; radiotherapy).

5 Bone malignancy (lymphoma; leukaemia; multiple myeloma; bones metastases).

Microcytic anaemia:

1 Iron-deficiency anaemia.

2 Thalassaemia (suspect if MCV is ↓ and red cell count is ↑).

3 Sideroblastic anaemia.

4 CT disorders (SLE; RA).

5 Anaemia of chronic disease (sometimes).

6 Aluminium toxicity (secondary to haemodialysis).

Iron-deficiency anaemia:

1 Poor diet.

2 Malabsorption.

3 Blood loss: GI[4] blood losses d/t worm infestation (ankylostomiasis), peptic ulcer, GI malignancy, haemorrhoids, fissure-in-ano; non-GI blood losses, e.g. haemoptysis, menorrhagia, etc.

---

1   In CT disorders (SLE; RA), cells are either normocytic or microcytic.

2   Aplastic anaemia – cells are either normocytic or macrocytic. Suspect, if besides ↓ Hb, TLC is ↓ or platelets are ↓.

3   Aplasia could be the first sign of leukaemia without any other marrow abnormality.

4   GI blood loss could be in the form of epistaxis, haematemesis, melaena, haematochezia or bleeding PR.

4 Multiple pregnancies.

Secondary iron overload:
1 Multiple blood transfusions.
2 Haematologic pathology (β-thalassaemia; aplastic anaemia; sideroblastic anaemia).
3 Liver pathology (chronic hepatitis B/C; alcoholic cirrhosis).

Macrocytic anaemia:
1 With megaloblastic bone marrow:
    a Folic acid/B_{12} deficiency.
    b Antifolate drugs (like phenytoin; methotrexate; azathioprine; hydroxyurea).
2 With normoblastic bone marrow:
    a Alcoholic liver disease.
    b Pregnancy.
    c Alcoholism.
    d Hypothyroidism.
    e Reticulocytosis.
3 With associated haematological disease:
    a Haemolytic anaemia ($\rightarrow$ reticulocytosis $\rightarrow \uparrow$ MCV).
    b Aplastic anaemia.
    c Myelophthisic anaemia (i.e. bone marrow infiltration).
    d Myelodysplastic syndromes (cytopenia, monocytosis, dysplastic morphology).
    e Myeloproliferative disorders.

It could be normocytic in haemolytic anaemia, aplastic anaemia, myelophthisic anaemia and hypothyroidism.

Vitamin B_{12} deficiency:
1 Nutritional deficiency – poor diet.
2 Malabsorption:
    a Gastric disease (pernicious anaemia; total gastrectomy).
    b Terminal ileal disease (Crohn's disease; ileocaecal TB; resection).
    c Infestation (*Diphyllobothrium latum*).
    d Bacterial infection (blind loop syndrome; diverticulosis).

Folic acid deficiency:
1 Poor diet.
2 Malabsorption.
3 $\uparrow$ requirement (pregnancy; haemolytic anaemia).
4 Drugs (methotrexate; pyrimethamine).

Microcytic anaemia – lab findings:

Test	Iron-deficiency	Chronic inflammation	Thalassaemia	Sideroblastic anaemia
RBC Morphology	Microcytic hypochromic.	Microcytic hypochromic or normal.	Microcytic hypochromic + target cells.	Variable.
Serum Iron	$\rightarrow$	$\rightarrow$	N or $\uparrow$	N or $\uparrow$
Ferritin	$\rightarrow$	N or $\uparrow$	N or $\uparrow$	N or $\uparrow$
TIBC	$\uparrow$	$\rightarrow$	N	N
Hb pattern	N	N	Abnormal	N

Tests for malabsorption:
1 Of fats:
  a Fat globules in the stools after special staining.
  b Faecal fat estimation.
  c ^{14}C triolein breath test.
2 Of carbohydrates:
  a Xylose absorption test.
  b Lactose tolerance test.
  c Hydrogen breath test with lactose.
3 Of proteins:
  a Nitrogen content of the stools.
  b Serum albumin level ($\downarrow$ level in the absence of hepatorenal disease or protein-losing enteropathy may indicate protein malabsorption).

Tests for bacterial colonisation of the small intestine:
1 Hydrogen breath test with lactulose.
2 ^{14}C glycocholic acid breath test.
3 Culture of jejunal aspirate.

Haemolytic anaemia:
1 Something is wrong with the RBCs (haemoglobinopathies, e.g. sickle-cell anaemia,[5] hereditary spherocytosis,[6] thalassaemia; G6PD deficiency; malaria [rupture of schizonts causes haemolysis]).
2 Antibodies develop against RBCs (warm/cold autoimmune haemolytic anaemia; Rhesus incompatibility [haemolytic disease of the newborn]; ABO mismatch blood transfusion).
3 RBCs suffer physical trauma (prosthetic heart valves; microangiopathic haemolytic anaemia).
4 Hypersplenism.

Warm antibodies[7] autoimmune haemolytic anaemia:
1 Idiopathic.
2 Lymphoma; leukaemia (CLL).
3 SLE.
4 Drugs (α-methyldopa).

Cold antibodies[8] autoimmune haemolytic anaemia:
1 Infection (infectious mononucleosis; *Mycoplasma pneumoniae* infection).
2 Lymphoma; leukaemia.

---

5 ↑ Hb S.
6 Autosomal dominant.
7 IgG antibodies attach to the RBCs at 37°C/ 98.6°F.
8 IgM antibodies attach to the RBCs below 37°C/ 98.6°F.

Findings in haemolysis:
1 $\uparrow$ reticulocyte index.
2 $\uparrow$ unconjugated bilirubin.
3 $\uparrow$ LDH.
4 $\downarrow$ or absent serum haptoglobin.
5 Haemosiderinuria (in cases of moderate haemolysis).[9]
6 Haemoglobinuria (in cases of severe haemolysis).

G6PD deficiency (X-linked recessive) – precipitated by:
1 Infection.
2 Drugs:
   a Analgesics.
   b Antibiotics (antimalarials; sulfonamides; chloramphenicol; nitrofurantoin).

Thalassaemia:

α-thalassaemia:
1 Mild form – not much disability.
2 Severe form – incompatible with life.

β-thalassaemia:
1 Thalassaemia minor (heterozygous) $\rightarrow \uparrow$ Hb A_2.
2 Thalassaemia major/Cooley's anaemia (homozygous) $\rightarrow \downarrow$ Hb A and $\uparrow$ Hb F.

$\uparrow$ Reticulocyte count:
1 RBCs rupture (haemolysis).
2 RBCs are lost (haemorrhage).
3 One week after B_{12} replacement therapy in a case of B_{12} deficiency anaemia.

Sideroblastic anaemia:
1 Congenital (X-linked).
2 Acquired:
   a Idiopathic (as one of the myelodysplastic disorders).
   b Uncommonly, secondary to chemotherapy, irradiation, lead/alcohol excess or anti-TB drugs.

Thrombocytopenic purpura:
1 Idiopathic thrombocytopenic purpura (ITP).
2 Secondary thrombocytopenic purpura:

---

9 Haemosiderinuria and haemoglobinuria are only seen in intravascular haemolysis.

a $\downarrow$ platelet synthesis (B_{12}/folate deficiency; bone marrow suppression/ infiltration).
b $\uparrow$ platelet destruction (hypersplenism; DIC; SLE).
c Massive blood transfusion.
d Drugs (sulfonamides; heparin; cytotoxics).

Disseminated intravascular coagulation (DIC):
1 Severe trauma.
2 Septicaemia.
3 Malignancy.
4 Obstetric conditions (eclampsia; abruptio placentae; intrauterine death of the foetus; amniotic fluid embolism).

RBC morphology – acanthocytosis (RBCs show spicules on the cell surface):
1 Abetalipoproteinaemia.

RBC morphology – anisocytosis:
1 Iron-deficiency anaemia.
2 Thalassaemia.
3 Megaloblastic anaemia.

RBC morphology – basophilic RBC stippling (d/t denatured RBCs indicating either defective Hb synthesis or accelerated erythropoiesis):
1 Lead poisoning.
2 Liver disease.
3 Haemoglobinopathy, e.g. thalassaemia.
4 Megaloblastic anaemia.
5 Myelodysplastic syndrome.

RBC morphology – blasts (nucleated precursor cells):[10]
1 Bone marrow infiltration.
2 Myelofibrosis.

RBC morphology – burr cells (irregularly shaped cells):
1 Uraemia.

RBC morphology – elliptocytes:
1 Hereditary elliptocytosis.

RBC morphology – helmet cells and fragmented cells:
1 Microangiopathic haemolytic anaemia.

---

10 Not normally found in the peripheral blood.

RBC morphology – pencil cells:
1 Iron-deficiency anaemia (with hypochromic microcytes).

RBC morphology – poikilocytosis:
1 Iron-deficiency anaemia.
2 Thalassaemia.
3 Myelofibrosis.

RBC morphology – polychromasia (RBCs of different ages stain unevenly; younger are bluer owing to RNA); reticulocyte count is raised:
1 Young red cells (implies high reticulocyte count).
   a Haemorrhage.
   b Haemolysis.
   c Haematinic replacement (Fe, B_{12}, folate).
   d Marrow infiltration.

RBC morphology – reticulocytosis (normal range: 0.8–2% or $<85 \times 10^9$/L); reticulocytes are young, larger RBCs containing RNA:
1 Haemorrhage.
2 Haemolysis.
3 Haematinic replacement (Fe, B_{12}, folate).

Reticulocytosis $\rightarrow$ ↑ MCV and polychromasia.

RBC morphology – schistocytes (fibrin strands fill small vessels $\rightarrow$ intravascular haemolysis $\rightarrow$ fragmented RBCs called schistocytes):
1 Microangiopathic haemolytic anaemia (MAHA):
   a Septicaemia/DIC.
   b Malignant hypertension.
   c Prosthetic heart valve induced haemolysis.
   d Haemolytic uraemic syndrome (HUS).
   e Thrombotic thrombocytopenic purpura (TTP).
   f Pre-eclampsia/eclampsia.

RBC morphology – sickle cells:
1 Sickle-cell disease (sickle cells + target cells).

RBC morphology – spherocytes:
1 Hereditary spherocytosis.
2 Any cause of haemolysis (e.g. autoimmune haemolytic anaemia).

RBC morphology – target cells (also called Mexican hat cells):
1 Liver disease.
2 Hyposplenism/post splenectomy.

3 Thalassaemia.

4 Iron-deficiency anaemia (in small numbers).

RBC morphology – tear drops:
1 Myelofibrosis.

Dimorphic picture (two populations of RBCs seen):
1 Mixed deficiency ($\downarrow$ Fe with $\downarrow$ B_{12} or folate).
2 After treatment of iron, folate or B_{12} deficiency.
3 After transfusion.
4 Primary sideroblastic anaemia (where, besides normal erythropoiesis, a clone of abnormal erythroblasts produces abnormal RBCs).

Howell–Jolly's bodies (RBC DNA nuclear remnants, which are normally removed by the spleen):
1 Post splenectomy.
2 Hyposplenism.
3 Dyserythropoietic states (e.g. megaloblastic anaemia; myelodysplasia).

Hyposplenism:
1 Congenital asplenism/splenectomy.
2 Sickle-cell anaemia.
3 GI diseases (e.g. coeliac disease, IBD).
4 Myeloproliferative disease.
5 Amyloidosis.

Left shift of neutrophils:
1 Immature cells are released into the general circulation from the marrow, e.g. in infection.

Right shift of neutrophils (presence of hypermature white cells, e.g. hypersegmented polymorphs [>5 lobes to nucleus]):
1 Megaloblastic anaemia.
2 Uraemia.
3 Liver disease.

Leucoerythroblastic anaemia (immature cells, e.g. myelocytes, pro-myelocytes, metamyelocytes and normoblasts seen in the peripheral film):
1 Myelofibrosis.
2 Bone marrow infiltration ($\rightarrow$ immature cells are displaced):
   a Tumour (primary; secondary).
   b Osteopetrosis (marble bone disease).
   c Storage disease.
3 Severe haemolysis.

4 Severe illness (major trauma; septicaemia; TB).

5 Leukaemoid reaction secondary to severe infection.

6 Storage disorders, e.g. Gaucher's disease.

7 Anorexia.

Leukaemoid reaction (marked leucocytosis: TLC >50 × 10⁹/L):

1 Burns.

2 Infection.

3 Leukaemia.

Pappenheimer's bodies (granules of siderocytes containing iron):

1 Lead poisoning.

2 Post splenectomy.

3 Carcinomatosis.

Heinz's bodies/'bite cells':[11]

1 G6PD deficiency.

Erythrocytosis:

1 Primary:

   a Polycythaemia vera.

2 Secondary:

   a Pathologic increase in erythropoietin (hypernephroma; ADPKD; transplant kidney; phaeochromocytoma; hepatoma; ovarian fibroma; cerebellar haemangioblastoma [part of von Hippel–Lindau's syndrome]).

   b $\downarrow O_2$ in blood → physiologic increase in erythropoietin (high altitude; lung pathology; smoking [carboxyhaemoglobin]; cyanotic heart disease).

Rouleaux formation (→ ↑ ESR):

1 Chronic inflammation.

2 Myeloma.

3 Paraproteinaemia.

Extravascular haemolysis (in the spleen):

1 RBCs are at fault (spherocytosis; haemoglobinopathies).

2 Hypersplenism.

3 Trauma.

---

11 On passing through the spleen, Heinz bodies may be removed, leaving an RBC with a 'bite' taken out of it.

Neutrophilia (normal count: 40–75% of white cells; 2–7.5 × 10⁹/L):

1 Bacterial infections.
2 Inflammation (e.g. MI; PAN).
3 Myeloproliferative disorders.
4 Disseminated malignancy.
5 Drugs (e.g. steroids).
6 Stress (e.g. trauma; haemorrhage; burns; surgery; seizures).

Neutropenia:

1 Infections (TB; viral infections).
2 ↓ production (aplastic anaemia; lymphoma; leukaemia).
3 ↑ destruction (hypersplenism, e.g. Felty's syndrome; megaloblastic anaemia; neutrophil antibodies, e.g. SLE, haemolytic anaemia).
4 Severe sepsis.
5 Iatrogenic:
   a Radiotherapy.
   b Drugs (carbimazole; anticonvulsants; antibiotics [chloramphenicol]; sulfonamides; NSAIDs [phenylbutazone]; cytotoxics).
6 Alcoholism.

Lymphocytosis (normal count: 20–45% of white cells; 1.5–4.5 × 10⁹/L):

1 Acute viral infections.
2 Chronic infections, e.g. TB; hepatitis; brucella; syphilis.
3 Leukaemias and lymphomas (especially CLL).

Atypical lymphocytes:

1 Viral infections (EBV [→ infectious mononucleosis[12]]; CMV; HIV; dengue; parvovirus).
2 Toxoplasmosis.
3 Typhus.
4 Leukaemias/lymphomas.
5 Lead poisoning.
6 Drug hypersensitivity.

Lymphopenia:

1 Iatrogenic (steroid therapy; post chemotherapy; radiotherapy).
2 SLE.
3 Legionnaires' disease.
4 Uraemia.
5 Infection (HIV).
6 Malignancy (marrow infiltration).

---

12 EBV (a DNA herpes virus) infection of B-lymphocytes → proliferation of T cells ('atypical' mononuclear cells), which are cytotoxic to EBV-infected cells.

Eosinophilia (normal count: 1–6%; 0.04–0.4 × 10⁹/L):

1 Allergies (e.g. atopic eczema; atopic asthma; Löffler's syndrome/pulmonary eosinophilia[13]).
2 Skin diseases: eczema; psoriasis; dermatitis herpetiformis; pemphigus drug reactions: erythema multiforme.
3 Parasitic infections.
4 During the convalescent phase of any infection.
5 Chronic infection (e.g. PAN).
6 Malignancy (lymphomas; eosinophilic leukaemias).
7 Adrenal insufficiency.

Monocytosis:

1 Iatrogenic: post chemo- or radiotherapy.
2 Chronic infections: TB; malaria; protozoa; brucellosis.
3 Malignancy: Hodgkin's disease; M4 and M5 AML; myelodysplasia.

Basophilia:

1 Urticaria.
2 Hypothyroidism.
3 Chronic inflammation: RA.
4 Viral infections.
5 Myeloproliferative disorders.

Bleeding disorders:

1 Defects of blood vessels.
2 Platelet disorders.
3 Clotting disorders.
4 DIC (consumptive coagulopathy).
4 Drugs.

Bleeding disorders – defects of blood vessels:

1 Acquired vasculopathy/vascular purpura:
  a Senile changes.
  b Meningococcal infection.
  c Septicaemia.
  d Scurvy.
  e Uraemia.
  f Henoch–Schönlein's purpura.
2 Congenital vasculopathy:
  a Hereditary haemorrhagic telangiectasia.
  b Osler–Weber–Rendu's syndrome.

---

13 Allergens (e.g. ascaris, ankylostoma; strongyloides; sulphonamides; hydralazine; nitrofurantoin) exposure → allergic infiltration of the lungs by eosinophils. CXR: diffuse fan-shaped shadowing. Rx: steroids + eradicate the underlying cause.

Bleeding disorders – platelet disorders:
1 Thrombocytopenia:
  a Idiopathic thrombocytopenic purpura (ITP).
  b Secondary thrombocytopenic purpura:
    i   Aplastic anaemia.
    ii   Marrow infiltration.
    iii Megaloblastic anaemia.
    iv Hypersplenism.
    v   Massive blood transfusion.
    vi DIC.
    vii Drugs – cytotoxics; sulfonamides; heparin.
2 Thrombocythaemia.
3 Thromboasthenia (normal number; defective function):
  a CML.
  b Renal failure.
  c Aspirin/NSAIDs therapy.
  d Glanzmann's disease (a rare hereditary disease).

Bleeding disorders – clotting disorders:
Hereditary:
1 Haemophilia A (X-linked recessive): PT normal; TT normal; APTT $\uparrow$; BT normal.
2 Haemophilia B (X-linked recessive): ditto.
3 von Willebrand's disease (autosomal dominant): PT normal; TT normal; APTT $\uparrow$; BT $\uparrow$.

Acquired:
1 Advanced liver disease.
2 Vitamin K deficiency: PT $\uparrow$; rest normal.
3 Heparin therapy: all increased (BT $\uparrow$ if platelet count is low).
4 DIC: ditto.

Differentiation between haemophilia A, B and von Willebrand's disease:
1 PT is normal and APTT $\uparrow$ in all three.
2 Whereas BT and Ristocetin platelet aggregation are normal in both HA and HB, in von Willebrand's disease Ristocetin platelet aggregation is $\downarrow$ and BT $\uparrow$.
3 Factor VIIIc is $\downarrow\downarrow$ in HA, $\downarrow$ in von Willebrand's disease and normal in HB.
4 Factor VIIVWB is $\downarrow$ in von Willebrand's disease alone.

Bleeding disorders – DIC (consumptive coagulopathy):
1 Obstetric conditions (dead foetus in utero; abruptio placentae; amniotic fluid embolism; eclampsia).
2 Malignancy.

3 Severe trauma.

4 Septicaemia.

Bleeding disorders – drugs:

1 Aspirin/NSAIDs.

2 Warfarin.

3 Steroids.

HELLP syndrome:

1 Haemolysis.

2 Elevated liver enzymes.

3 Low platelets.

Management of HELLP:

1 Intravenous corticosteroids in females <34 weeks gestation to defer delivery.

2 Attempt delivering the foetus ASAP.

3 If having seizures → magnesium sulphate.

4 If hypertensive → antihypertensives.

5 If bleeding → blood and platelets transfusion.

6 If renal functions are deteriorating → dialysis.

Complications of hereditary haemorrhagic telangiectasia (HHT):

1 CNS: seizures; migraine; TIA/CVA; cerebral abscess.

2 Chest: haemothorax; haemoptysis; pulmonary HTN.

3 GI: haemorrhage.

4 Haematological: iron-deficiency anaemia (d/t blood loss); polycythaemia (d/t chronic hypoxia).

8 Nephrology

Pre-renal oliguria/anuria:
1 ↓ renal perfusion (hypovolaemic[1]/cardiogenic/septic shock).
2 Hepatorenal syndrome.

Pre-renal failure vs. acute tubular necrosis (ATN):
1 Urine output: low in both.
2 Urine osmolality: >500 in pre-renal failure; <350 in ATN.
3 U/P osmolality ratio: 1.5:1 in pre-renal failure; 1.1:1 in ATN.
4 U/P creatinine ratio: >20:1 in pre-renal failure; <20:1 in ATN.
5 Urea/creatinine ratio: >20:1 in pre-renal failure; <20:1 in ATN.
6 Urine Na^+: <20 mmol/L in pre-renal failure; >50 mmol/L in ATN.
7 Fractional Na^+ excretion:[2] <1 in pre-renal failure; >1 in ATN.
8 Urine sediment: normal in pre-renal failure; cellular debris in ATN.

Renal oliguria/anuria:
1 Vascular pathologies (total occlusion of renal artery/vein; vasculitis [SLE; PAN; scleroderma]; acute glomerulonephritis).
2 Tubular pathologies:
   a ATN:
      i   ↓ renal perfusion.
      ii Pigments (e.g. haemoglobin – haemoglobinuria d/t haemolysis, myoglobin – rhabdomyolysis).
      iii Drugs like PCM; aminoglycosides; heavy metals; radiocontrast agents.
   b Intratubular deposition:
      i   Gout (uric acid deposition).
      ii Multiple myeloma (paraproteins deposition).
3 Interstitial nephritis:
   a Drug-induced:
      i   NSAIDs.
      ii Antibiotics (penicillins; cephalosporins; sulfonamides). Diuretics (loop and thiazides).
   b Infections (streptococcal; legionella; leptospirosis).
   c Granulomatous disease (sarcoidosis).
4 CRF patients: acute or chronic.

---

1   D/t vomiting, diarrhoea, haemorrhage, burns.
2   It is the most sensitive index.

Post-renal oliguria/anuria:
1 Obstructive uropathy (stones; tumour; BOO; prostatomegaly – benign or malignant).

Anuria:
1 Shock → ATN → anuria.
2 Rapidly progressive glomerulonephritis.
3 Total renal artery/vein occlusion.
4 Total urinary tract obstruction.

Components of nephritic syndrome:
1 Haematuria.
2 Azotaemia.
3 HTN.

Reversible causes of renal failure:
1 Dehydration.
2 UTI.
3 Obstructive uropathy.
4 Metabolic ($\downarrow K^+$; $\uparrow Ca^{2+}$; $\uparrow$ uric acid [usually >15 mg/dL]).
5 CVS (CHF; HTN).
6 Nephrotoxic drugs.

Complications of ARF:
1 Metabolic acidosis.
2 Fluid overload.
3 Electrolyte abnormalities ($\downarrow Na^+$; $\uparrow K^+$; $\downarrow Ca^{2+}$; $\uparrow Mg^{2+}$; $\uparrow PO_4^{3-}$).

Nocturia:
1 BPH.
2 DM.
3 CRF.
4 LVF/CCF.

Renal manifestation of NSAIDs:
1 ATN.
2 Acute interstitial nephritis.
3 Minimal change GN.

Chronic renal failure (CRF):
1 Chronic glomerulonephritis.
2 Bilateral chronic pyelonephritis.
3 Diabetic/hypertensive nephropathy.

4 Obstructive uropathy (stones; tumour; BOO;[3] benign/malignant prostatic enlargement).
5 Drugs (painkillers; heavy metals).
6 Vasculitis (SLE; PAN: scleroderma).
7 Hypercalcaemia.

Chronic kidney disease with 'normal-sized' kidneys:
1 ADPKD.
2 Diabetes mellitus.
3 Amyloidosis.
4 Multiple myeloma.

Signs of end-stage renal disease:
1 Pruritus.
2 Muscular twitching/fits.
3 Drowsiness/coma.
4 Uraemic smell on the breath.
5 Hiccough/vomiting.
6 Hypotension.
7 Kussmaul's respiration.
8 Pericardial rub.

Differentiation b/w ARF and CRF:
1 Anaemia,[4] non-concentrated urine, $\downarrow Ca^{2+}$, $\uparrow PO_4^{3-}$ and small shrunken
   kidneys: all common in CRF; rare or absent in ARF.
2 Renal osteodystrophy: late feature of CRF; absent in ARF.
3 Proteinuria: uncommon in ARF; rare in CRF.

Bone changes in renal osteodystrophy:
1 Osteomalacia (d/t dihydroxycholecalciferol).
2 Osteitis fibrosa cystica (d/t secondary hyperparathyroidism).
3 Osteosclerosis.

Resistance to erythropoietin in CKD patients:
1 Iron, folic acid or vitamin B_{12} deficiency.
2 Blood loss.
3 Inadequate dialysis.
4 Chronic inflammation/sepsis.
5 Aluminium toxicity.
6 Severe hyperparathyroidism.

---

3   BOO: bladder outlet obstruction.

4   May occur in ARF, if secondary haemorrhage.

Renal failure in multiple myeloma:
1 Renal infiltration of plasma cells/intratubular precipitation of paraproteins.
2 Amyloidosis.
3 Hyperviscosity → renal vein thrombosis.
4 Dehydration.
5 Metabolic (hypercalcaemia; hyperuricaemia).
6 Infection (immunoparesis → recurrent pyelonephritis).
7 Iatrogenic (NSAIDs therapy for pain relief).

Palpable kidney:
Bilateral:
1 Bilateral hydronephrosis/pyonephrosis.
2 ADPKD.

Unilateral:
1 Unilateral hydronephrosis/pyonephrosis.
2 Malignancy (renal cell ca. in adults; Wilm's tumour in children).
3 Compensatory hypertrophy if contralateral kidney is small or absent.

Coloured urine:
1 Haematuria/haemoglobinuria/myoglobinuria.
2 Obstructive jaundice.
3 Porphyria.
4 Alkaptonuria.
5 Drugs (rifampicin).
6 Beetroot.

Haematuria:
1 Glomerulonephritis.
2 Papillary necrosis (NSAIDs; DM; sickle-cell anaemia).
3 Stones[5]/infection[6]/tumour of any structure of the urinary tract from kidneys till urethra.
4 Menstruation.
5 Systemic disease (SLE; PAN; infective endocarditis).
6 Trauma.
7 Bleeding disorder.

Gross haematuria: urine is red in colour.

Microscopic haematuria: urine is of normal colour. On microscopy, 2–5 RBCs/HPF are seen.

---

5   Renal; ureteric; vesicular.

6   Pyelonephritis; renal TB; cystitis; prostatitis; urethritis.

Painful haematuria:
1 UTI.
2 Renal/ureteric calculus.
3 Trauma (Foley catheterisation; recent painful sexual intercourse).

Painless haematuria:
1 Glomerulonephritis.
2 UTI.
3 Tumour (renal/ureteric/bladder).
4 Systemic disease (SLE; PAN; infective endocarditis).
5 Bleeding disorder.
6 Sickle-cell anaemia.
7 Malignant hypertension.

Proteinuria:
1 Postural/orthostatic proteinuria.[7]
2 Non-specific febrile illness.
3 UTI.
4 Glomerulonephritis d/t any cause ($\rightarrow$ nephritic/nephrotic syndrome).

Urinary casts – hyaline casts:
Not indicative of renal disease:
1 After strenuous exercise.
2 Concentrated urine.
3 Diuretic therapy.
4 Febrile illness.

Urinary casts – red cell casts:
1 GN.

Urinary casts – white cell casts:
Indicative of infection/inflammation:
1 Pyelonephritis.
2 Interstitial nephritis.

Urinary casts – renal tubular cell casts:
1 ATN.
2 Interstitial nephritis.

Urinary casts – coarse granular casts:
1 Non-specific (e.g. may be d/t ATN).

---

7   May be found in an ambulant young person. Early morning specimen fails to show proteinuria.

Urinary casts – broad waxy casts:
1 Indicative of stasis in enlarged collecting tubules:
2 CRF.

Isolated urinary incontinence (no faecal incontinence):
1 UTI.
2 Prostatism.
3 Uterine prolapse.
4 Weakness of pelvic floor muscles.

Incontinence of urine and faeces:
1 Neurogenic bladder (associated with UMN- or LMN-type paraparesis).
2 Faecal impaction with overflow.
3 CNS pathology (epileptic fits; severe depression; dementia).

Polyuria/polydipsia:
Solute diuresis – urine osmolality >300 mOsm/L
(urine osmolality > plasma osmolality):
1 Diabetes mellitus.
2 Diuretic therapy/diuretic phase of ARF.
3 Electrolyte imbalances ($\downarrow$ K$^+$; $\uparrow$ Ca^{2+})

Water diuresis – urine osmolality <250 mOsm/L
(urine osmolality < plasma osmolality):
1 $\uparrow$ water content of the urine (d/t diabetes insipidus or compulsive polydipsia).

Isothenuria
(urine osmolality = plasma osmolality):
1 CRF.

Plasma (P) and urinary (U) Na$^+$ and osmolality in various conditions:
1 Diabetes insipidus: (P) Na$^+$/osm $\uparrow$ or normal; (U) Na$^+$/osm $\downarrow$.
2 SIADH: (P) Na$^+$/osm $\downarrow$; (U) Na$^+$/osm $\uparrow$.
3 Hypoadrenalism: same as SIADH.
4 Hypothyroidism: same as SIADH.
5 Effective volume depletion:[8] (P) Na$^+$/osm $\downarrow$ or normal; (U) Na$^+$ $\downarrow$; (U) osm $\uparrow$.
6 Water intoxication: everything is $\downarrow$.

---

8   It includes dehydration from GI losses, excessive perspiration, CCF and hypoalbuminaemic states (CLD; nephrotic syndrome). An exception is renal failure d/t interstitial nephritis in which Na$^+$ excretion is increased even in the presence of dehydration.

Polydipsia + polyuria + respiratory involvement:
1 Diabetes insipidus.

Hyperkalaemia:
1 Metabolic acidosis (renal failure; DKA; salicylate poisoning).
2 Addison's disease.
3 Drugs (oral or IV K^+ administration; K^+-sparing diuretics; ACEI).
4 Recent blood transfusion.
5 Spurious result d/t haemolysis in the specimen bottle.[9]

Hypokalaemia:
1 Excessive loss of water (diuretic therapy;[10] vomiting; diarrhoea; purgative abuse; intestinal fistula; ileostomy; villous adenoma of rectum).
2 Excessive mineralocorticoid activity (Conn's syndrome [primary hyper-aldosteronism]; Cushing's syndrome).
3 Renal tubular acidosis (RTA).
4 Drugs (diuretics; β-agonists).

Hypernatraemia:
1 Hypertonic plasma with hypervolaemia (e.g. excess IV saline).
2 Hypertonic plasma with hypovolaemia (e.g. polyuria in diabetes mellitus/ insipidus).
3 Primary hyperaldosteronism (Conn's syndrome (d/t adrenal hyperplasia/ tumour.

Hyponatraemia:[11]
1 Dehydration (net loss of Na^+ and H_2O).
2 Dilutional hyponatraemia (H_2O gain; no net loss of Na^+):
   a CCF.
   b Cirrhosis of liver.
   c Nephrotic syndrome.
   d Syndrome of inappropriate ADH (SIADH) secretion.[12]

SIADH:
1 CNS pathology (head injury; meningitis; encephalitis; SOL [haematoma; abscess; tumour]; GB syndrome).
2 Chest infection (legionella pneumonia; empyema; TB).

---

9   Normal K^+ when repeated with no delay in delivery to the lab.

10 It is the commonest cause of hypokalaemia.

11 Na^+ <120 mmol/L → symptoms of ↓ Na^+ commence owing to brain cell oedema; Na^+ <110 mmol/L → severe symptoms.

12 Suspect SIADH, if serum Na^+ level is <130 mmol/L, urine osmolality >300 mOsm/kg and urine osmolality > plasma osmolality despite plasma osmolality being low (<270 mmol/kg).

3 Malignancy (oat cell ca; thymoma; ca. pancreas).
4 Acute intermittent porphyria.
5 Drugs (opiates; carbamazepine; chlorpromazine; chlorpropamide; vincristine).

Hypercalcaemia:
1 Endocrinopathies (primary/tertiary hyperparathyroidism; hyperthyroidism; ectopic PTH from ca. lung; acromegaly; Addison's disease; phaeochromocytoma).
2 Bone disease (multiple myeloma; lymphoma; leukaemia; bone metastases[13]).
3 Drugs (e.g. vitamin D intoxication; thiazide diuretics).
4 Sarcoidosis.
5 Milk–alkali syndrome.

Hypocalcaemia:
1 Renal pathology (chronic renal failure): $\downarrow Ca^{2+}$; $\pm \uparrow PO_4^{3-}$; $\pm \uparrow$ alkaline phosphatase; $\pm \uparrow$ creatinine; normochromic normocytic anaemia.
2 Vitamin D deficiency/resistance: $\downarrow Ca^{2+}$; $\downarrow PO_4^{3-}$; $\pm \uparrow$ alkaline phosphatase; $\downarrow 1,25(OH)2$ vitamin D.
3 Pancreatic pathology (acute pancreatitis): $\downarrow Ca^{2+}$; $\downarrow$ or normal PO_4^{3-}; normal alkaline phosphatase; $\uparrow$ serum amylase.
4 Parathyroid pathology:
   a Hypoparathyroidism[14] (following thyroidectomy/parathyroidectomy/radiations; autoimmune; congenital [DiGeorge syndrome]).
   b Pseudohypoparathyroidism (peripheral resistance).[15]
1 Drugs (e.g. calcitonin).
2 Rhabdomyolysis.[16]
3 Fluid overload: $\downarrow Ca^{2+}$; $\downarrow PO_4^{3-}$; normal alkaline phosphatase.

Hypocalcaemia – clinical features:
1 Symptoms:
   a Sensory: paraesthesias; circumoral numbness.
   b Motor: cramps; tetany (carpopedal spasms).
   c Can progress to convulsions, laryngeal stridor or psychosis.
2 Signs:
   a Chvostek's sign.
   b Trousseau's sign.

---

13 From ca. thyroid, breast, lung, kidney, colon, ovary.
14 $\downarrow Ca^{2+}$; $\pm \uparrow PO_4^{3-}$; PTH $\downarrow$ or normal.
15 Short stature, obesity, round face, short metacarpals, $\downarrow$ or normal Ca^{2+}, $\uparrow$ PTH, $\pm \uparrow PO_4^{3-}$.
16 $\uparrow Ca^{2+}$ is deposited in the damaged muscle tissue $\rightarrow \downarrow$ serum Ca^{2+}; $\uparrow PO_4^{3-}$; $\uparrow\uparrow$ CPK; $\pm \uparrow$ creatinine.

↓ Ca²⁺ and ↑ PO₄³⁻:
1 CRF.
2 Parathyroid pathology (hypoparathyroidism; pseudohypoparathyroidism).
3 Hypomagnesaemia (d/t peripheral resistance to PTH).
4 Rhabdomyolysis.

Hyperphosphataemia:
1 Renal failure.
2 Endocrinopathy (hypoparathyroidism; acromegaly).
3 ↑ intake of vitamin D/phosphate.
4 Tumour lysis syndrome.

Hypophosphataemia:
1 IV glucose/TPN.
2 Recovery phase of DKA.
3 Endocrinopathy (primary hyperparathyroidism).
4 Vitamin D deficiency.
5 Renal tubular disease.

Hypermagnesaemia:
1 Magnesium infusion/enema/oral overdose.
2 Renal failure.
3 Adrenal insufficiency.
4 Milk–alkali syndrome.
5 Drug-induced (theophylline toxicity; lithium).

Nephrotic syndrome – diagnostic features:
1 Generalised oedema.
2 Urine protein excretion >3.5 g/24 hr.
3 Hypoalbuminaemia (albumin <3 g/dL).

Nephrotic syndrome – causes:
1 Vascular pathology (glomerulonephritis;[17] vasculitis [secondary to SLE, etc]; microangiopathy secondary to diabetes mellitus).
2 Amyloidosis.
3 Infection (*Plasmodium malariae*).
4 Malignancy (lung).
5 Drugs (disease modifying antirheumatic drugs, e.g. penicillamine, gold, etc).

Membranous glomerulonephritis:
1 Chronic infection (hepatitis B; malaria; syphilis).

---

17 Minimal change GN; membranous GN; proliferative GN; focal segmental glomerulosclerosis.

2 Malignancy (lymphoma; CLL; ca. lung/stomach/colon).
3 Drug-induced (NSAIDs; captopril; penicillamine; gold).
4 CT disorders (SLE; RA; MCTD; Sjögren's syndrome).
5 Sarcoidosis.
6 PBC.
7 GB syndrome.

Focal segmental glomerulosclerosis:
1 HIV/AIDS.
2 Small-vessel vasculitis (Churg–Strauss's syndrome and Wegener's granulomatosis).

Mesangioproliferative GN/IgA nephropathy/Berger's disease:[18]
1 Coeliac disease/dermatitis herpetiformis.
2 Cirrhosis of liver.
3 Mycosis fungoides (cutaneous T-cell lymphoma).
4 Wiskott–Aldrich's syndrome.

Mesangiocapillary GN (MCGN):
1 Familial.
2 Partial lipodystrophy (C3 nephritic factor).
3 Sickle-cell anaemia.
4 RA.
5 α1-antitrypsin deficiency.
6 Kartagener's syndrome.
7 Shunt nephritis.[19]

Rapidly progressive GN (crescentic GN):
1 SLE.
2 Vasculitis (ANCA +ve or –ve).
3 Goodpasture's syndrome.

GN and hypocomplementaemia:
1 Primary complement deficiency.
2 Cryoglobulinaemia type 2.
3 SLE.
4 GN (poststreptococcal; mesangiocapillary).
5 Endocarditis.
6 Shunt nephritis.

---

18 Precipitated by URTI.

19 Staphylococcal infection of the ventriculo-atrial shunt.

CT disorders with renal involvement:
1 SLE.
2 Sjögren's syndrome.
3 Systemic sclerosis.
4 RA.
5 MCTD.

Drug-induced GN:
1 NSAIDs.
2 Captopril.
3 DMARDs (penicillamine; gold) – cause membranous GN.

↑ **Creatinine:**
1 ↑ production: large muscle mass; rhabdomyolysis.
2 ↓ tubular secretion: drug-induced (K^+ -sparing diuretics; trimethoprim; aspirin; cimetidine).
3 Non-creatinine chromogen (ketoacidosis).

↓ **Creatinine:**
1 ↓ production:
   a Physiologic decrease in muscle mass (advanced age).
   b Pathologic decrease in muscle mass (cachexia).
   c Liver disease ($\rightarrow$ ↓ hepatic creatinine synthesis).
2 Dilution: pregnancy; ↑ ADH.

↑ **Urea:**
1 ↑ production: high protein diet; catabolic state (e.g. GI bleed; steroid therapy); sepsis.
2 ↓ excretion: pre-renal failure d/t hypovolaemic/cardiogenic shock; ATN; post-renal failure; CRF.
3 Drugs: corticosteroids; tetracyclines.

↓ **Urea:**
1 ↓ production: liver disease; starvation.
2 Dilution: pregnancy; SIADH.
3 Sickle-cell anaemia.

Rhabdomyolysis:
1 Muscle injury:
   a RTA.
   b Strenuous exercise (marathon running).
   c Burns/electrocution.
   d Hypothermia.
   e Status epilepticus.

f   Neuroleptic malignant syndrome.
g   Septicaemia.
h   Drugs (statins; amphetamines).

↑ CPK:

1   Physiological in blacks (up to 300 IU/L).
2   Muscle pathology (trauma; polymyositis; muscular dystrophy; statins/fibrates).
3   Endocrinopathy (hypothyroidism).
4   Infection (septicaemia; leptospirosis).

Glomerulonephritis after sore throat:

1   Poststreptococcal GN.[20]
2   IgA nephropathy.[21]

ARF + C3 nephritic factor positive:

1   Mesangiocapillary glomerulonephritis (MCGN) type II.

ARF + ASOT + anti-DNAse or antihyaluronidase positive:

1   Poststreptococcal GN.

ARF + blood culture positive:

1   May be secondary to bacterial endocarditis.

ARF + ↓ complement:

1   SLE.
2   Postinfectious GN (poststreptococcal GN; bacterial endocarditis).
3   Mixed essential cryoglobulinaemia.
4   MCGN type I and II.

ARF + ↑ complement:

1   Systemic vasculitis.

ARF + ↑ polyclonal immunoglobulins:

1   SLE.
2   Sarcoidosis.
3   Postinfectious.

---

20 Throat culture and ASO titre positive; haematuria occurs 10 days after sore throat; recurrent haematuria or haematuria after six months is rare.

21 Throat culture and ASO titre negative; haematuria occurs five days after sore throat; recurrent haematuria and haematuria occur commonly after six months.

ARF + ↑ monoclonal immunoglobulins:
1 Multiple myeloma.

ARF + ↑ IgE:
1 Churg–Strauss's syndrome.

ARF + ↑ IgA:
1 Henoch–Schönlein's purpura.
2 IgA nephropathy.

ARF + ↑ CRP:
1 ↑ in most cases but not usually in SLE.

ARF + neutrophilia and thrombocytosis:
1 Systemic vasculitis.

ARF + eosinophilia:
1 Rapidly progressive glomerulonephritis.
2 Drug-induced tubulo-interstitial nephritis.
3 Churg–Strauss's syndrome.
4 Cholesterol micro-emboli.

ARF + lymphopenia:
1 SLE.

ARF + thrombocytopenia:
1 SLE.
2 Drug-induced interstitial nephritis.

Minimal change glomerulonephritis:
1 Autoimmune.
2 Hypersensitivity (cow's milk allergy; bee-sting reaction).
3 Drugs (NSAIDs; pamidronate; lithium).
4 Malignancy (Hodgkin's lymphoma).

GN + ANCA + asthma + eosinophilia:
1 Churg–Strauss's syndrome.

GN + ANCA + respiratory granulomas:
1 Wegener's granulomatosis.

GN + ANCA + systemic vasculitis:
1 Microscopic polyangiitis.

GN + ANCA + no extrarenal disease:
1 ANCA-associated crescentic GN.

GN + anti-GBM + lung haemorrhage:
1 Goodpasture's syndrome.

GN + anti-GBM + no lung haemorrhage:
1 Anti-GBM GN.

GN + ANA:
1 Lupus GN.

GN + IgA:
1 IgA nephropathy.

GN + antipathogen antibodies:
1 Postinfectious or peri-infectious GN.

GN + cryoglobulins:
1 Cryoglobulinaemic GN.

GN + C3 nephritic factor:
1 Membranoproliferative GN.

GN + light microscopy findings:
1 Diffuse proliferative GN: poststreptococcal GN.
2 Mesangioproliferative GN: IgA nephropathy (Burger's disease and Henoch–Schönlein's purpura).
3 Crescentic GN: rapidly progressive GN.

GN + immunofluorescence microscopy findings:
1 IgG + C3 – granular pattern + (diffuse proliferative GN on light microscopy): poststreptococcal GN.
2 IgA (± IgG, C3) + (mesangioproliferative GN on light microscopy): IgA nephropathy (Burger's disease and Henoch–Schönlein's purpura).
3 IgA + IgG + C3 (granular pattern) + (crescentic GN on light microscopy): rapidly progressive GN (d/t LE, mixed cryoglobulinaemia, subacute infective endocarditis, shunt infection).
4 IgG + C3 (linear pattern) + (crescentic GN on light microscopy): rapidly progressive GN (d/t Goodpasture's syndrome or idiopathic).
5 No immunoglobulins + (crescentic GN on light microscopy): rapidly progressive GN (d/t Wegener's granulomatosis, PAN or idiopathic).
6 No immunoglobulins ± mesangial proliferation: minimal change GN.
7 IgM and C3 in sclerotic segments + (focal segmental sclerosis on light

microscopy): focal segmental GN.

8 Granular IgG and C3 along capillary loops + (thickened GBM and spikes on light microscopy): membranous GN.

9 IgG, IgM, granular C3, C1q and C4 + (↑ mesangial cells and matrix and splitting of GBM on light microscopy): membranoproliferative GN type I (associated with URTI).

10 C3 + (↑ mesangial cells and matrix and splitting of GBM on light microscopy): membranoproliferative GN type II.

GN + electron microscopy:

1 Subepithelial deposits: poststreptococcal GN.

2 Mesangial deposits: IgA nephropathy (Burger's disease and Henoch–Schönlein's purpura).

3 Widening of GBM + (crescentic GN on light microscopy): rapidly progressive GN (d/t Goodpasture's syndrome or idiopathic).

4 No deposits + (crescentic GN on light microscopy): rapidly progressive GN (d/t Wegener's granulomatosis, PAN or idiopathic).

5 Deposits in subepithelium, subendothelium or mesangium + (crescentic GN on light microscopy): rapidly progressive GN (d/t LE, mixed cryoglobulinaemia, subacute infective endocarditis, shunt infection).

6 Fusion of foot processes: minimal change GN; focal segmental GN.

7 Dense deposits in subepithelial area: membranous GN.

8 Dense deposits in subendothelial area: membranoproliferative GN type I.

9 Dense deposits in GBM: membranoproliferative GN type II.

Indications of renal biopsy in a child with heavy proteinuria:

1 Non-response to conventional therapy/frequent relapses.

2 Obvious evidence of multisystem vasculitis.

3 Presence of red cells/casts in the urine.

Linear IgG deposition along the glomerular basement membrane:

1 Anti-GBM disease (Goodpasture's syndrome).

2 SLE.

3 Diabetes mellitus.

Acid–base balance:

- pH <7.35 = acidosis (metabolic/respiratory).
- pH >7.45 = alkalosis (metabolic/respiratory).
- If pH, $PaCO_2$ and HCO_3^- all go in one direction (↑ or ↓) = metabolic pathology.
- If pH goes in one direction (↑ or ↓) and $PaCO_2$ and HCO_3^- in another = respiratory pathology.
- After determining that it is metabolic/respiratory, acidosis/alkalosis, calculate anion gap and then excess anion gap.

- Anion gap = serum $(Na^+ + K^+) - (Cl^- + HCO_3^-)$.
- Excess anion gap (EAG) = anion gap $- 12 + HCO_3^-$.
- If EAG <23 = non-anion gap, metabolic acidosis (typical of all renal tubular acidosis).
- If EAG >30 = metabolic acidosis.

pH <7.4 (acidosis) + PaCO$_2$ >40 mmHg:
1 Respiratory acidosis (pH ↓ + PaCO2 ↑ + HCO3– ↑; compensatory response = ↑ renal HCO3– reabsorption).

Respiratory acidosis:
1 Hypoventilation d/t any cause (obesity; respiratory muscle paresis/paralysis; thoracic cage deformities).
2 COPD/acute attack of asthma.
3 Drugs (opioids; sedatives).

pH <7.4 (acidosis) + PaCO$_2$ <40 mmHg:
1 Metabolic acidosis with compensation (pH ↓ + PaCO2 ↓ + HCO3– ↓; compensatory response = hyperventilation).

Two categories of metabolic acidosis:
1 Metabolic acidosis with ↑ anion gap (>12 mEq/L).[22]
2 Metabolic acidosis with normal anion gap (8–12 mEq/L)

Metabolic acidosis with ↑ anion gap:[23]
MUDPILES
1 **M**ethanol.
2 **U**raemia.
3 **D**KA.
4 **P**araldehyde.
5 **I**ron tablets/INH.
6 **L**actic acidosis.
7 **E**thylene glycol/methylene poisoning.
8 **S**alicylic acid poisoning.

Metabolic acidosis with normal anion gap (8–12 mEq/L):
1 Fluid loss (severe diarrhoea; pancreatic fistula; ureterosigmoidostomy).
2 Hyperchloraemia.
3 Renal tubular acidosis.
4 Glue sniffing.
5 Acetazolamide therapy.

---

22 Occurs because of the addition of 'acid' and 'unmeasured anions' to the body.

23 Anion gap = $(Na^+ + K^+) - (Cl^- + HCO_3^-)$.

pH >7.4 (alkalosis) + PaCO₂ <40 mmHg:
1 Respiratory alkalosis (pH ↑ + PaCO2 ↓ + HCO3– ↓; compensatory response = renal HCO3– secretion).

Respiratory alkalosis:
1 Hyperventilation d/t CNS stimulation:
   a Anxiety.
   b Hypoxia.
   c Aspirin ingestion (early).
   d CNS pathology (encephalitis; brainstem injury).
2 Hyperventilation d/t pulmonary pathology:
   a Pneumonia.
   b Pulmonary embolism.
   c Pulmonary oedema.
   d Asthma.
   e Lung fibrosis.

pH >7.4 (alkalosis) + PaCO₂ >40 mmHg:
1 Metabolic alkalosis with compensation (pH ↑ + PaCO2 ↑ + HCO3– ↑; compensatory response = hypoventilation).

Metabolic alkalosis:
1 Vomiting.
2 Diuretic use.
3 Antacid use.
4 Hyperaldosteronism.

Combined respiratory and metabolic acidosis:
1 Acute LVF.
2 Massive pulmonary embolism.
3 Aspirin poisoning.
4 Acute exacerbation of COPD (→ diuretics prescribed to relieve pulmonary congestion → dehydration → pre-renal failure).
5 Pneumonia (legionnaires' disease) → septicaemia → renal failure.
6 ARF → fluid overload.
7 Septicaemia d/t any cause complicated by ARF and ARDS.
8 Malaria complicated by pneumonia.
9 Renal pulmonary syndromes (anti-GBM disease; Wegener's granulomatosis; PAN).

Renal tubular acidosis (RTA) type 1 (distal):
1 Inherited.
2 Acquired:
   a Liver pathology (chronic active hepatitis; PBC).

   b Renal pathology (obstructive nephropathy).
   c Vitamin D intoxication.
   d Drugs (tetracycline).

RTA type 1 (distal) – complications:
1 Hypercalciuria ($\rightarrow$ nephrocalcinosis; calculi).
2 UTIs.
3 Growth retardation.

RTA type 2 (proximal):
1 Inherited (part of Fanconi's syndrome),
2 Acquired:
   a Hyperparathyroidism.
   b Multiple myeloma.
   c Drugs (acetazolamide).
   d Poisoning (lead; arsenic).

RTA type 2 (proximal) – effects:
Proximal tubular dysfunction $\rightarrow$ $\downarrow$ reabsorption thus $\uparrow$ excretion of multiple agents:
1 Glycosuria.
2 Aminoaciduria.
3 Phosphaturia.
4 Uricosuria.

RTA type 2 (proximal) – complications:
1 Osteomalacia (excretion of phosphate)/rickets.
2 Fanconi's syndrome.

Long-term complications of dialysis:
1 Anaemia.
2 Renal pathology (renal osteodystrophy; acquired cystic disease).
3 Vascular disease.
4 Amyloidosis.
5 Aluminium toxicity (rare).

Indications of nephrectomy prior to transplantation:
1 ADPKD.
2 Uncontrolled HTN.
3 UTI.
4 Renal or urothelial malignancy (must be over two years recurrence-free prior to transplantation).

HLA antigens:
Mnemonic: DR-BAC
1 DR.
2 B.
3 A.
4 C.

HLA antigens – importance of HLA matching in renal transplantation:
Mnemonic: DR-BAC
1 DR > B > A > C.

Renal transplantation – good/acceptable match:
Good match:
- No DR + no or only one B mismatch.

Acceptable match:
- One DR **or** one B mismatch.

Renal pathologies which can recur following transplantation:
1 All glomerulonephritides can recur (especially focal segmental glomerulosclerosis; IgA nephropathy; membranous GN; mesangiocapillary GN).
2 Vasculitis (monitor autoimmune antibodies, e.g. anti-DNA; ANCA).
3 Alport's syndrome.[24]

---

24 Alport's syndrome: anti-GBM disease + sensorineural deafness + lenticonus.

9 Endocrinology

Hyperaldosteronism:
Primary:
  1 Conn's syndrome.
  2 Bilateral adrenal hyperplasia.
  3 Glucocorticoid-remediable aldosteronism (GRA).[1]

Secondary ($\downarrow$ renal perfusion $\to$ $\uparrow$ renin $\to$ $\uparrow$ aldosterone):
  1 Cirrhosis of liver.
  2 CCF.
  3 Accelerated HTN.
  4 Diuretics.
  5 Renal artery stenosis.
  6 Bartter's syndrome.[2],[3]

HTN + hypokalaemia:
  1 Diuretic therapy.
  2 Primary hyperaldosteronism.
  3 Secondary hyperaldosteronism d/t renal artery stenosis.

Hypokalaemic metabolic alkalosis ($\downarrow$ K$^+$; $\downarrow$ H$^+$; $\uparrow$ HCO$_3^-$):
  1 $\uparrow$ GI loss of K$^+$:[4]
   a Villous adenoma.
   b Laxative abuse.
  2 $\uparrow$ renal loss of K$^+$:[5]
   a Diuretic abuse.
   b Cushing's syndrome (especially secondary to ectopic ACTH production).
   c Primary/secondary hyperaldosteronism.
   d Bartter's syndrome.

---

1   GRA = ACTH $\to$ aldosterone release. Its treatment is dexamethasone 1 mg/day PO $\to$ $\downarrow$ ACTH $\to$ $\downarrow$ aldosteronism.

2   Whereas patients of Bartter's syndrome remain normotensive, hypertension develops in cases of primary hyperaldosteronism.

3   Bartter's syndrome $\to$ hypokalaemic hypochloraemic metabolic alkalosis.

4     $\uparrow$ GI loss of K$^+$ $\to$ hypokalaemia $\to$ 24-hr urinary K$^+$ <20 mmol.

5   24-hr urinary K$^+$ >20 mmol.

Goitre:
1 Sporadic.
2 Endemic (iodine deficiency).
3 Pregnancy.
4 Autoimmune thyroid disease.
5 Thyroiditis.
6 Drug-induced (ATDs*; lithium; amiodarone).

*ATDs: antithyroid drugs.

↑ Thyroid-binding globulin – TBG (→ ↑ total T3/T4 and normal free T3/T4):
1 Oestrogen-containing OCPs.
2 Pregnancy.[6]
3 Liver pathology (hepatitis A; chronic active hepatitis; PBC; acute intermittent porphyria).

↓ TBG (→ ↓ total T3/T4 and normal free T3/T4):
1 Androgens or steroids therapy/Cushing's syndrome.
2 Hypoproteinaemia (malabsorption; cirrhosis of liver; nephrotic syndrome).
3 Active acromegaly.
4 Any severe systemic illness.

Drugs displacing T4/T3 from TBG:
1 Phenytoin.
2 Aspirin.
3 Frusemide.

Myxoedema:
1 Congenital (dyshormonogenesis).
2 Thyroiditis (Hashimoto's thyroiditis; spontaneous atrophic thyroiditis).
3 Iatrogenic (antithyroid drugs; radioiodine therapy; thyroidectomy).

Thyrotoxicosis:
1 Primary hyperthyroidism:
  a Graves' disease.
  b Toxic multinodular goitre.
  c Toxic adenoma.
2 Secondary hyperthyroidism:
  a TSH-secreting pituitary adenoma.

---

6 Since free T4 and T3 levels remain normal in pregnancy, it should not be confused with thyrotoxicosis, in which free T4 level is high (↑ T3 in T3 toxicosis) with suppressed TSH. Serum TSH level decreases in the 1st trimester.

    b   Thyroid hormone resistance syndrome ($\uparrow$ TSH and $\uparrow$ free T4 and free T3).

3 Thyrotoxicosis without hyperthyroidism:
    a   Thyroiditis (subacute [de Quervain's]; silent and postpartum; drug-induced [amiodarone]).
    b   Excess intake of thyroxine.
    c   Ectopic thyroid tissue: struma ovarii (teratoma containing functional thyroid tissue).

Thyroid hormone concentrations in various thyroid conditions:
Raised free T4 and T3:
1 Primary hyperthyroidism: $\uparrow\uparrow$ free T4; $\uparrow$ free T3; undetectable TSH.
2 T3 toxicosis: normal free T4; $\uparrow\uparrow$ free T3; undetectable TSH.
3 Subclinical hyperthyroidism: normal free T4 and T3; $\downarrow$ or undetectable TSH.
4 Secondary hyperthyroidism (TSHoma): $\uparrow$ free T4 and T3; $\uparrow$ or normal TSH.
5 Thyroid hormone resistance: $\uparrow$ free T4 and T3; $\uparrow$ or normal TSH.

Low free T4 and T3:
1 Primary hypothyroidism: $\downarrow$ free T4; $\downarrow$ or normal free T3; $\uparrow$ TSH.
2 Secondary hypothyroidism: $\downarrow$ free T4; $\downarrow$ or normal free T3; $\downarrow$ or normal TSH.

Atypical TFT[7] – suppressed TSH and normal free T4:[8]
1 T3 toxicosis (approximately 5% of thyrotoxicosis).
2 Subclinical hyperthyroidism.

Atypical TFT – suppressed TSH and normal free T4 and free T3:
1 Early subclinical thyrotoxicosis.
2 Recovery from thyrotoxicosis.
3 Excess thyroxine replacement.

Atypical TFT – detectable TSH and elevated free T4 and free T3:
1 TSH-secreting pituitary tumour (TSHoma).
2 Pituitary thyroid hormone resistance syndrome.
3 Heterophile antibodies.

Atypical TFT – elevated free T4 and low free T3:
1 Amiodarone therapy.

---

7   TFTs: thyroid function tests.
8   In thyrotoxicosis, free T4 is high and TSH suppressed.

Sick euthyroid syndrome (non-thyroidal illness syndrome) – ↓ T4 and T3; normal or ↓ TSH:
1 Starvation.
2 Any severe illness (ITU; severe infection; renal/hepatic/cardiac failure; end-stage malignancy).

Drugs that cause hypothyroidism:
1 Antithyroid drugs (carbimazole; propylthiouracil; radioactive iodine).
2 Lithium.[9]
3 Amiodarone.

Complications of hypothyroidism:
1 CVS (IHD; pericardial effusion).
2 CNS (myxoedema madness;[10] myxoedema coma).
3 Hypothermia.

Antithyroid antibodies in Graves' disease:
1 TSH receptor antibody (stimulating): 70–100%.
2 Antithyroid peroxidase (anti-TPO): 70–80%.
3 Anti-thyroglobulin: 30–50%.

Antithyroid antibodies in Hashimoto's thyroiditis:
1 TSH receptor antibody (blocking): 10–20%.
2 Antithyroid peroxidase (anti-TPO): majority of the cases.
3 Anti-thyroglobulin: majority of the cases.

Radionuclide scan appearance in thyroid disease:
1 Graves' disease: enlarged gland; ↑ homogeneous radionuclide uptake.
2 Toxic nodule: a solitary area of ↑ uptake.
3 Thyroiditis (e.g. de Quervain's): low or absent uptake.
4 Thyrotoxicosis factitia:[11] ↓ uptake.
5 Thyroid carcinoma: cancerous tissue requires an adequate level of TSH for 131I uptake. TSH levels can be raised by withholding T3 10 days before radionuclide scan or by giving recombinant TSH injection prior to scanning.

---

9 Thyroid function tests should be checked periodically (six-monthly) in all patients on lithium or amiodarone therapy.

10 Frank psychosis with hallucinations and delusions.

11 Thyrotoxicosis factitia: thyroxine use in non-thyroidal disease: clinically there is no thyroid enlargement; ↑ free T4; ↓ TSH; ↓ radionuclide uptake; ↓ thyroglobulin – this differentiates thyrotoxicosis factitia from thyroiditis (which shows ↓ radionuclide uptake but ↑ thyroglobulin).

Thyroid nodule:
1 Colloid nodule.
2 Cyst.
3 Lymphocytic thyroiditis.
4 Benign tumour (Hurthle cell; follicular).
5 Malignant tumour (papillary; follicular).

Thyroidectomy – complications:
1 Immediate:
  a Recurrent laryngeal nerve palsy.
  b Thyroid crisis.
  c Hypoparathyroidism.
  d Local haemorrhage (→ laryngeal compression).
  e Wound infection.
1 Late:
  a Hypothyroidism.
  b Keloid formation.

MEN-I (chromosome 11):
Mnemonic: PPP
1 **P**arathyroid.
2 **P**ancreas (insulinoma; gastrinoma; glucagonoma; VIPoma; PPPoma).
3 **P**ituitary (60% prolactinoma).

MEN-IIA (chromosome 10):
1 Parathyroid.
2 Thyroid (medullary carcinoma thyroid – MCT).
3 Phaeochromocytoma.

MEN-IIB:
1 Parathyroid.
2 Thyroid (medullary carcinoma thyroid – MCT).
3 Phaeochromocytoma.
4 Mucosal neuromas.
5 Marfanoid.

Contents of cavernous sinus:
1 Cranial nerves III, IV, V (ophthalmic branch) and VI.
2 Internal carotid artery.
3 Sympathetic fibres (that surround the artery).

↑ Prolactin:
1 Dopamine antagonists (metoclopramide; phenothiazines).
2 Oestrogen-containing OCPs.

3 Endocrinopathy (prolactinoma; hypothalamic/pituitary stalk lesion; hypothyroidism; PCOS).
4 Coitus/pregnancy/lactation (nipple suckling).
5 Stress; chest wall trauma.
6 Renal or hepatic failure.

↓ Prolactin:
1 Dopamine.
2 Dopamine agonists (bromocriptine).

Growth hormone deficiency:
1 Pituitary pathology:
  a Infection (abscess; TB).
  b Tumour.
  c Infarction (post-traumatic bleed into the gland and bleed into the tumour are the causes).
2 Parapituitary tumour (craniopharyngioma).

Panhypopituitarism:
1 SOL (pituitary or extrapituitary).
2 Iatrogenic (irradiation; surgery).
3 Sheehan's syndrome.
4 Pituitary apoplexy.
5 Infiltrative disorder (haemochromatosis; lymphocytic hypophysitis).

Cushing's syndrome:
1 Steroid therapy.
2 ↑ ACTH production (pituitary tumour; ectopic ACTH production by lung malignancy).
3 Adrenal tumour.

Cushing's disease – dexamethasone suppression test interpretation:
1 Full suppression = physiological.
2 Some suppression = pituitary-dependent disease.
3 No suppression = ectopic ACTH/adrenal tumour.

Addison's disease:
1 Autoimmune destruction.
2 TB.
3 Adrenal haemorrhage/infarction (Waterhouse–Friderichsen's syndrome).
4 Metastases (from ca. lung).

Addison's disease vs. panhypopituitarism:

1 Whereas low Na$^+$ is common in both, high K$^+$ only occurs in Addison's disease.
2 Hyperpigmentation occurs only in Addison's disease.

Congenital adrenal hyperplasia (CAH) – autosomal recessive:

- 21-hydroxylase deficiency → ↓ mineralocorticoid, ↓ corticosteroid production and ↑ androgen production (all precursors are driven into androgen production → virilisation; genital ambiguity).

Mild 21-hydroxylase deficiency:

1 Ovarian pathology (PCOS).
2 Adrenal pathology (Cushing's syndrome; androgen-secreting adrenal tumour).

Precocious puberty:
Gonadotrophin-dependent (↑ FSH and LH):

1 Idiopathic.
2 CNS problem (head injury; CNS infection; cerebral tumour; hydrocephalus).
3 Iatrogenic (head and neck surgery/irradiation).

Gonadotrophin-independent (normal FSH and LH):

1 CAH.
2 Adrenal/ovarian tumour.
3 Exogenous androgen/oestrogen therapy.
4 Severe hypothyroidism.
5 Von Recklinghausen's syndrome.
6 McCune–Albright's syndrome.

Delayed puberty:

1 Constitutional (idiopathic delay in the activation of HPO axis).
2 Overt or occult severe systemic disease (e.g. starvation, anorexia nervosa, severe asthma, cystic fibrosis, etc).
3 Primary hypogonadism (ovarian failure) – most commonly d/t Turner's syndrome; others include Klinefelter's, Noonan's and androgen insensitivity, etc.
4 Rarely secondary hypogonadism (hypothalamus/pituitary failure) – d/t pituitary chromophobe adenoma; craniopharyngioma; Laurence–Moon–Biedl's syndrome).

Hypogonadism in males:

1 Gonadotrophin failure:
  a Hypopituitarism.

   b Hyperprolactinaemia ($\rightarrow$ hypopituitarism).
2 Primary gonadal disease:
   a Congenital (undescended testes; Klinefelter's syndrome).
   b Acquired (testicular torsion; castration; radiotherapy; renal/hepatic failure).

Hypogonadism in females:
1 Gonadotrophin failure:
   a Hypothalamic–pituitary disease.
   b Kallman's syndrome.
2 Complete ovarian failure:
   a Dysgenesis; Turner's syndrome; Swyer's syndrome.[12]
   b Autoimmune oophoritis; oophorectomy/radiotherapy/chemotherapy.
3 Partial ovarian failure:
   a PCOS.
   b Resistant ovary syndrome.
4 Adrenal pathology: 17α-hydroxylase deficiency.
5 Iatrogenic: cytotoxic drug therapy.

Gynaecomastia:
Physiological:
1 Neonate; puberty; elderly; obesity.

Pathological:
1 Endocrinopathy (hyper- or hypothyroidism; acromegaly).
2 CLD ($\rightarrow$ $\downarrow$ oestrogen metabolism).
3 Neoplasia:
   a Oestrogen-secreting adrenal or testicular tumour.
   b HCG-secreting lung or testicular tumour.
   c Carcinoma breast.
4 Chromosomal problem (Klinefelter's syndrome).
5 Drugs:
   a Oestrogen; gonadotrophins.
   b Digoxin.
   c Spironolactone.
   d Cimetidine.
   e Cyproterone.
   f Cannabis/high alcohol intake.

---

12 Phenotypically female; XY karyotype; gonadal dysgenesis with high incidence of gonadoblastoma.

Absent pubic hair:
1 Hypogonadism.
2 Hypopituitarism.

Male-distribution pubic hair in a female:
1 Male-hormone-secreting adrenal tumour (adrenal virilism).

Female-distribution pubic hair in a male:
1 Cirrhosis of liver.

Characteristics of PCOS (Stein–Leventhal's syndrome):
1 Irregular menstruation.
2 Impaired fertility.
3 Obesity; hirsutism; acne.
4 ↓ oestradiol level; ↑ oestrone level; testosterone level slightly >3 nmol/L.
5 LH slightly ↑; FSH slightly ↓; LH/FSH ratio generally >2.

Secondary diabetes mellitus:
1 Pancreatic pathology (chronic pancreatitis; ca. pancreas; pancreatectomy; haemochromatosis; cystic fibrosis).
2 Insulin antagonists (acromegaly; thyrotoxicosis; pregnancy; Cushing's syndrome; phaeochromocytoma).

Diabetic ketoacidosis (DKA): diagnostic features:
1 Hyperglycaemia >250–600 mg/dL (13.9–33.3 mmol/L).
2 Serum osmolality 300–320 mOsm/mL.
3 pH 6.8–7.3.
4 Serum bicarbonate <15 mEq/L.
5 Anion gap – ↑.
6 Arterial pCO_2 – 20–30 mmHg.
7 Serum ketones ++++.

DKA – causes:
1 Discontinuation of insulin.
2 Infection (URTI; LRTI; UTI).
3 Infarction (coronary; cerebral).
4 Surgery.

Hyperglycaemic hyperosmolar state (HHS)[13] – diagnostic features:
1 Hyperglycaemia 600–1200 mg/dL (33.3–66.6 mmol/L).
2 Serum osmolality 330–380 mOsm/mL.
3 pH >7.3.

---

13 Previously called HONK (hyperosmolar non-ketotic).

4 Serum bicarbonate >15 mEq/L (often normal or slightly ↓).

5 Anion gap – normal or slightly ↑.

6 Arterial PCO2 – normal.

7 Serum ketones ±.

Hyperglycaemic hyperosmolar state (HSS)[14] – causes:

1 Discontinuation of oral antidiabetic drugs.

2 Infection (URTI; LRTI; UTI).

3 Infarction (coronary; cerebral).

4 Surgery.

Lactic acidosis – diagnostic features:

1 Severe acidosis with hyperventilation.

2 Blood pH <7.30.

3 Serum bicarbonate <15 mEq/L.

4 Anion gap >15 mEq/L.

5 Absent serum ketones.

6 Serum lactate >5 mmol/L.

Lactic acidosis – causes:

1 Shock (hypovolaemic; septic).

2 ↓ oxygen supply to the tissues (shock; severe anaemia; CO poisoning).

3 Organ failure (hepatic/renal).

4 Bowel infarction.

5 Infection (complication of malaria).

6 Malignancy (leukaemia).

7 Drug-induced (metformin therapy).

8 TPN.

9 G6PD deficiency.

Hypoglycaemia – diagnostic features:

1 Blood glucose <40 mg/dL with a serum insulin level of 6 μU/mL or more.

2 Recovery is often immediate upon glucose administration.

Hypoglycaemia – causes:

In diabetics:

1 Overdose of glucose-lowering drugs (insulin; oral hypoglycaemics).

2 Missed meals.

3 Unaccustomed exercise.

---

14 Plasma osmolality = $2 \times (Na^+ + K^+)$ + blood sugar (mmol/L) + urea (mmol/L) – normal = 285–295 mOsm/kg. Sugar: 1 mmol/L = 18 mg/dL; Urea: 1 mmol/L = 6 mg/dL; Na^+/K^+: 1 mEq/L = 1 mmol/L.

Unrelated to diabetes:

1 Alcoholism.
2 Post gastrectomy.
3 Endocrinopathies:
   a Addison's disease.
   b Hypothyroidism.
   c ↑ insulin (d/t insulinoma; ↓ insulin metabolism [in severe liver/ renal disease]; exogenous insulin administration; ↑ insulin-like growth factor [IGF] secretion by retroperitoneal fibrosarcoma or mesothelioma).
4 Organ failure (pituitary; adrenal; hepatic; renal).
5 Sepsis.
6 Reactive hypoglycaemia.

Goals in diabetes mellitus to prevent complications:

1 30 minutes of aerobic exercise five times a week → achieve BMI 28.
2 BP ≤130/80 mmHg.
3 Hb A1c ≤7%.
4 Total cholesterol ≤5 mmol/L.
5 LDL cholesterol ≤2.3 mmol/L.

Diabetes mellitus – acute complications:

1 DKA.
2 HONK.
3 Lactic acidosis.
4 Hypoglycaemia.

Diabetes mellitus – chronic complications:

1 Microvascular:
   a Eye (diabetic retinopathy; early cataract).
   b Diabetic nephropathy.
   c Diabetic neuropathy.
2 Macrovascular:
   a CVA.
   b IHD.
   c PVD.
3 Others:
   a ↑ risk of infections (carbuncle; moniliasis; pneumonia; TB; diabetic foot).
   b Skin: necrobiosis lipoidica diabeticorum (NLD) – lipodystrophy d/t insulin injections.

Diabetic neuropathy:

1 Polyneuropathy: bilaterally symmetrical, glove and stocking distribution, mixed (mainly sensory), peripheral neuropathy.

2 Mononeuropathy: 3rd and 6th cranial nerves; ulnar, median, sciatic or common peroneal nerves.

3 Autonomic neuropathy:[15] postural hypotension; gastroparesis; nocturnal diarrhoea; constipation; faecal/urinary incontinence; impotence.

4 Diabetic amyotrophy: painful weakness and wasting of quadriceps muscle.

Interpretation of GTT:

	BSF in mmol/L*	BSF in mg/dL*
Normal	<6.1	<110
Diabetes mellitus	>7.0	>125
Impaired fasting glucose (IFG)	6.1–7.0	110–125
Gestational diabetes	>5.8	>105
*1 mmol/L glucose = 18 mg/dL		

	2 hr PP* in mmol/L	2 hr PP* in mg/dL
Normal	<7.8	<140
Diabetes mellitus	>11.1	>200
Impaired glucose tolerance (IGT)	7.8–11.1	140–200
Gestational diabetes	>6.7	>120
Abbreviations: *PP = postprandial (after oral administration of 75 g glucose)		

Transient glycosuria: one blood glucose level b/w fasting and 2 hr post-prandial is >180 mg/dL, which becomes normal at 2 hr. It is also called intestinal or lag-storage glycosuria. The cause is either rapid absorption of glucose from the gut (secondary to partial gastrectomy or thyrotoxicosis) or defective storage of glucose in the liver (secondary to any liver disease).

---

15 Painless MI/peptic ulceration is common in this subgroup.

Glycosuria:
1 Diabetes mellitus.
2 Renal glycosuria.[16]

Flat glucose tolerance curve (plasma glucose levels fail to rise following an oral glucose load):
1 Physiological.
2 Malabsorption.
3 Endocrine pathology (hypopituitarism with secondary growth hormone deficiency; Addison's disease).

Diabetic retinopathy:
1 Background or simple retinopathy (not a threat to vision):
  a Microaneurysms (seen as 'dot' haemorrhages) + 'blot' haemorrhages + hard exudates (small, multiple, irregularly shaped exudates that are usually closely aggregated at one or more places).
2 Preproliferative retinopathy (not a threat to vision):
  a Features of background retinopathy + soft exudates (only 1 or 2, large fluffy exudates).
3 Proliferative retinopathy (a threat to vision):
  a Features of preproliferative retinopathy + new vessel formation (neo-vascularisation) + retinitis proliferans.

Advanced diabetic eye disease:
- Vitreous haemorrhage.
- Retinal detachment.
- Rubeotic glaucoma.

Diabetic maculopathy:
1 Loss of central vision (peripheral vision spared).
2 Macular oedema + macular stars (hard exudates arranged in a horseshoe or circular fashion around the macula).

Diabetic retinopathy – criteria for referral to an ophthalmologist:
1 Preproliferative/proliferative retinopathy.
2 Maculopathy.
3 Advanced diabetic eye disease.

Central (cranial) diabetes insipidus:
1 Idiopathic.
2 DIDMOAD syndrome.[17]

---

16 Glycosuria when RBS is within the normal range on GTT.

17 DIDMOAD syndrome: **d**iabetes **i**nsipidus; **d**iabetes **m**ellitus; **o**ptic **a**trophy; **d**eafness.

3 Pituitary pathology:
  a Infection (abscess; TB).
  b Tumour.
  c Infarction (post-traumatic bleed into the gland; bleed into the tumour).
  d Pituitary surgery.
4 Parapituitary tumour (craniopharyngioma).
5 Hypothalamic pathology (lymphocytic hypophysitis; hypothalamic infiltration [sarcoidosis, histiocytosis X]).

Nephrogenic diabetes insipidus:
1 Primary: X-linked/autosomal dominant ($\rightarrow$ childhood onset).
2 Secondary:
  a Electrolyte disturbance ($\downarrow K^+$; $\uparrow Ca^{2+}$).
  b Renal pathology (ADPKD; obstructive uropathy; chronic pyelonephritis; sarcoidosis).
  c Drug-induced (lithium; demeclocycline; glibenclamide; aminoglycosides; amphotericin).

Unexplained loss of weight:
Weight loss with good appetite:
1 Diabetes mellitus.
2 Thyrotoxicosis.
3 Worm infestation.
4 Malabsorption syndrome.

Weight loss with anorexia:
1 Malignancy.
2 Chronic inflammation (CT disorders).
3 Chronic infection (TB).
4 Chronic liver/renal disease.
5 Anaemia.
6 Psychogenic.

Obesity – (BMI >30 kgm^{-2}):
1 Simple obesity d/t overeating and sedentary life style (both limb and truncal obesity; TSH and fT4 normal; 24-hr urinary cortisol normal).
2 Hypothyroidism.
3 Pseudohypoparathyroidism (obesity + bone problem + $\downarrow Ca^{2+}$).
4 Cushing's syndrome.
5 Frohlich's syndrome (obesity + hypogonadism).
6 Laurence–Moon–Biedl's syndrome (obesity + hypogonadism + polydactyly).

Vitamin deficiency:
1 Vitamin A deficiency:
  a Protein-energy malnutrition (PEM).
2 Vitamin B1 (thiamine) deficiency:
  a Alcoholism.
  b Dietary restriction.
3 Vitamin B2 (riboflavin) deficiency:
  a PEM.
4 Niacin deficiency:
  a Alcoholism.
  b Carcinoid syndrome.
  c Iatrogenic (isoniazid therapy).
5 Vitamin B6 (pyridoxine) deficiency:
  a Iatrogenic (isoniazid; hydralazine).
6 Vitamin C deficiency:
  a Dietary deficiency.
7 Vitamin D deficiency:
  a Renal failure.
  b Dietary deficiency.
8 Vitamin E deficiency:
  a Fat malabsorption.
  b Abetalipoproteinaemia.
9 Vitamin K deficiency:
  a Biliary obstruction.
  b Antibiotic therapy.

False-positive sweat Na⁺ test:
1 Endocrinopathy (hypothyroidism; hypoparathyroidism; Addison's disease).
2 α1-antitrypsin deficiency.
3 Mucopolysaccharidosis.

10 Infectious diseases

Contraindications to vaccination:
1 Pregnancy: pregnancy should be avoided for up to one month after vaccination.
2 Concurrent illness: untreated malignancy; severe febrile illness.
3 Concurrent therapy: patient on immunosuppressive therapy.
4 Other live vaccine given within the last three weeks.

Bactericidal antibiotics:
1 Penicillins.
2 Cephalosporins.
3 Aminoglycosides.

Antibiotics – inhibitors of DNA replication:
1 Quinolones.
2 Metronidazole.

Antibiotics – inhibitors of folate synthesis:
1 Co-trimoxazole.

Antibiotics – inhibitors of protein synthesis:
1 Macrolides.
2 Aminoglycosides.
3 Tetracycline.
4 Chloramphenicol.
5 Clindamycin.
6 Fusidic acid.

Antibiotics – inhibitors of cell wall synthesis:
1 β-lactams:
   a Penicillins.
   b Cephalosporins.
   c Carbapenems (imipenem).
   d Monobactams (aztreonam).
2 Glycopeptides:
   a Vancomycin.
   b Teicoplanin.

Non-HIV antiviral drugs:
1 Acyclovir: active against HCV and VZV.
2 Ganciclovir: active against HCV, VZV and CMV.
3 Ribavirin: active against RSV, HCV (in combination with interferon therapy) and Lassa fever.

Antituberculous drugs – mechanisms of action:
1 Rifampicin: inhibits DNA replication by inhibiting RNA-polymerase.
2 Isoniazid: inhibits cell wall synthesis.
3 Ethambutol: inhibits bacterial RNA synthesis.
4 Pyrazinamide: not exactly known; probably works inside phagosomes.
5 Streptomycin: inhibits bacterial protein synthesis.

Antibiotics with urinary excretion (suitable in UTIs):
1 Trimethoprim/co-trimoxazole.
2 Ampicillin/co-amoxiclav.
3 Cephalexin.
4 Nalidixic acid.
5 Nitrofurantoin.

Encephalitis – aetiological agents:
1 Viral causes:
  a HSV (mostly type 1).
  b VZV.
  c Arboviruses (e.g. Japanese encephalitis).
  d Coxsackie virus.
  e EBV.
  f Echoviruses.
  g Enteroviruses.
  h HIV.
  i Rabies.
2 Toxoplasmosis.
3 African trypanosomiasis ('sleeping sickness').
4 Cysticercosis (pig/bovine tapeworms).

Meningitis – aetiological agents:
1 Viral:
  a Common: enteroviruses.
  b Less common: mumps; adenoviruses; HSV; VZV; HIV.
2 Bacterial:
  a Common: meningococci; pneumococci; *Haemophilus influenzae*.
  b Less common: *Staphylococcus aureus*; AFB; *Listeria monocytogenes*; leptospirosis; *Borrelia burgdorferi* (Lyme disease).
3 Fungal (almost always in immunocompromised): coccidioidomycosis; *Cryptococcus neoformans*.

4 Rickettsial (uncommon): Rocky Mountain spotted fever.

Acute bacterial meningitis in neonates:
1 Group B streptococci.
2 *E. coli.*

Chronic bacterial meningitis:
1 *Mycobacterium tuberculosis.*

Fever + headache + petechial/purpuric rash:
1 Meningococcal septicaemia.

Non-responding meningitis with no organism isolated in CSF:
Cause is infective, but:
1 Epidural abscess has formed.
2 Organism is resistant to antibiotics.
3 Unusual organism (will not respond to the 'routine' regimen).

Non-infective cause (neurosarcoidosis; malignancy).

Infections caused by *Chlamydia trachomatis*:
Males:
1 Non-gonococcal urethritis; prostatitis.
2 Epididymitis.
3 Proctitis (in homosexuals).
4 *Lymphogranuloma venereum.*
5 Reactive arthritis/Reiter's arthritis.

Females:
1 Non-gonococcal urethritis.
2 Cervicitis/PID.
3 Peri-hepatitis (Fitzhugh–Curtis' syndrome).

Neonates (vertical transmission):
1 Conjunctivitis.
2 Pneumonia.

Infections caused by *Chlamydophila pneumoniae*:
1 Pneumonia.

Infections caused by *Chlamydophila psittaci*:
1 Psittacosis.

Cellulitis – aetiological agents:
1 Common: *Streptococcus pyogenes*; *Staphylococcus aureus*.
2 Hospital-acquired: *Staphylococcus aureus*; MRSA; gram-negative bacilli.
3 In a diabetic: mixed infection (streptococci; staphylococci; gram-negative bacilli; anaerobes).
4 H/o saltwater injury: *Vibrio vulnificus*.
5 H/o freshwater injury: *Aeromonas hydrophila*.

Severe pneumonia – definition:
One or more of the following in a patient with clinical and/or radiological signs of pneumonia:
1 BP <90 mmHg systolic.
2 Respiratory rate >30/min.
3 Multilobar involvement on CXR.
4 ↓ O2: PaO2 <8.0 kPa (breathing room air).
5 ↑ urea >7 mmol/L.

Community-acquired pneumonia – aetiological agents:
1 Most common: *Streptococcus pneumoniae*.
2 Common: *Haemophilus influenzae*; *Mycoplasma pneumoniae*; *Chlamydophila pneumoniae*.
3 Less common: *Staphylococcus aureus*; *Legionella pneumophila*; influenza virus; *Chlamydophila psittaci*; *Coxiella burnetii*; *Moraxella catarrhalis*.

LRTI – causative organisms in immunocompromised:
1 Pseudomonas.
2 PCP.
3 Aspergillus.
4 CMV.

Simultaneous involvement of LRT and CNS:
1 Infection (streptococcal/staphylococcal pneumonia; atypical pneumonia [mycoplasma; legionnaires' disease]; TB; malaria; HIV; cysticercosis).
2 Malignancy (ca. lung).
3 Granulomatous disease (sarcoidosis; histiocytosis X).
4 Vasculitides (PAN; Wegener's granulomatosis; SLE).
5 Neuroectodermal syndromes (neurofibromatosis; tuberous sclerosis).
6 Sickle-cell syndrome.

Complications of mycoplasma pneumonia:
1 CNS: aseptic meningitis; encephalitis; transverse myelitis; GB syndrome; peripheral neuropathy.
2 CVS: myocarditis; pericarditis.
3 Haematological: cold antibodies autoimmune haemolytic anaemia; thrombocytopenia.

4 GIT: NVD.
5 Endocrine: SIADH.
6 Skin: EM; SJS; bullous myringitis.
7 Rheumatological: myositis; arthritis.

Vertebral osteomyelitis and discitis – aetiological agents:
1 Common (>50%): *Staphylococcus aureus*.
2 Less common:
   a IV drug abuser; antecedent h/o UTI: coliforms.
   b H/o infective endocarditis: streptococci.
   c Suggestive travel history: brucellosis.

Lymphadenopathy with a travel history:
1 TB.
2 Leishmaniasis.
3 Mycoses (coccidioidomycosis; histoplasmosis).
4 Trypanosomiasis.
5 Rickettsial disease.

IV drug abuser with fever and dyspnoea:
1 Cardiac pathology: right-sided endocarditis; cardiac failure (secondary to valvular incompetence).
2 Pulmonary pathology: pneumonia (community-acquired; aspiration); pulmonary embolism (right-sided endocarditis → septic emboli; femoral injections → DVT → pulmonary embolism).
3 Immunosuppression (HIV).

Fever + hypotension (shock) + confusion:
1 Toxic shock syndrome.
2 Meningococcal septicaemia.
3 Non-meningococcal septic shock (primary could be skin infection, LRTI, UTI, cholangitis, etc).

Normal respiratory rate (10–16/min):
1 Physiological.
2 Near death (d/t exhaustion).

Tuberculosis – risk factors:
1 Contact with a TB patient (usually a family member).
2 Alcoholic or IV drug abuser.
3 Immunosuppression (HIV; renal failure; immunosuppressive therapy).
4 Travel history to an endemic area.
5 Social history: homeless; overcrowding.

ICU patient with persistent unexplained fever with h/o multiple blood transfusion:
1 Viral infection (CMV; parvovirus) – leucopenia is suggestive.
2 Hepatitis – deranged LFTs suggestive.

Sore throat:
1 Viral infection:
  a Common: EBV; CMV; adenoviruses; enteroviruses.
  b Less common: HIV.
2 Bacterial infection:
  a Common: streptococci.
  b Less common: anaerobes; mycoplasma.

Sexually transmitted exudative pharyngitis:
1 *Neisseria gonorrhoeae*.

Sore throat + h/o recent travel to eastern Europe or a developing country:
1 Diphtheria.

Sore throat + thrombosis of the internal jugular vein + LRTI:
1 Lemierre's disease (caused by Fusobacterium necrophorum).

Viral sore throat – complications:
1 EBV: meningitis; encephalitis; GB syndrome.
2 Hepatitis (EBV; CMV).
3 Splenomegaly.
4 Haematological: haemolysis; leucopenia; ITP.
5 Rash.

Bacterial sore throat – complications:
1 Lemierre's disease (caused by *Fusobacterium necrophorum*).
2 Acute rheumatic fever.
3 Acute glomerulonephritis.
4 Skin (scarlet fever; guttate psoriasis).

Acute complications of malaria:
1 Cerebral malaria.
2 Pulmonary oedema (non-cardiac).
3 Hepatic failure.
4 Renal failure (*Plasmodium malariae* → nephrotic syndrome).
5 Blackwater fever.
6 Hypoglycaemia/lactic acidosis.
7 Malarial dysentery.
8 Abortion.

Chronic complications of malaria:
1 Tropical splenomegaly.
2 Malarial nephropathy.

Criteria for positive Widal test:[1]
1 Single titre[2] of 1:320 or higher.
2 Rising titre.

Early (1st week) complications of enteric fever (d/t septicaemia):
1 Meningitis.
2 Chest (pneumonitis; myocarditis).
3 Musculoskeletal (arthritis; osteomyelitis; periostitis; myositis).
4 Thrombophlebitis.

Late (3rd week) complications of enteric fever:
1 Ileal haemorrhage/perforation.
2 Cholecystitis/gallbladder perforation.
3 Chronic carrier.[3]

HIV-associated conditions:
Based on increasing immune deficiency, HIV patients are divided into three groups:
- Asymptomatic patients with persistent generalised lymphadenopathy.
- Symptomatic but don't have any condition included in group C – called AIDS-related complex (ARC).
- Patients with conditions meeting WHO 'case definition' of AIDS.

Each group is further divided into 1, 2 and 3 depending on the CD4 count (>500/µL; 200–499/µL; <200/µL respectively).

Features of HIV positive group B patients:
Symptoms:
1 Fever; weight loss.
2 Diarrhoea.
3 Fatigue; malaise.

---

1 Antibodies against 'O' antigen (somatic antigen) and not 'H' antigen (flagellar antigen) are significant and are checked in the Widal test.

2 'Titre' is the highest dilution of serum in which antibodies are detectable.

3 A person who continues to excrete the bacilli in the faeces one year after the infection is called a chronic carrier.

Signs:
1 Mouth (candidiasis; oral hairy leucoplakia).
2 Splenomegaly; lymphadenopathy.
3 Peri-anal herpes.
4 Wasting.

11 Clinical pharmacology

Hepatic cytochrome P$_{450}$ enzyme inducers:
1 Anticonvulsants (carbamazepine; phenytoin; phenobarbitone).
2 Antituberculous (rifampicin).
3 Antidiabetics (sulphonylureas).
4 Alcohol (chronic use)/smoking.

Important drugs whose metabolism is affected by enzyme inducers:
1 Warfarin ($\downarrow$ anticoagulant effect $\rightarrow$ $\downarrow$ INR).
2 OCP (failure $\rightarrow$ pregnancy).
3 Enzyme inducers decrease the therapeutic effects of each other.
4 Theophylline ($\downarrow$ effect).
5 Corticosteroids ($\downarrow$ effect).
6 Cyclosporine ($\downarrow$ immunosuppressive effect).

Hepatic cytochrome P$_{450}$ enzyme inhibitors:
1 Anticonvulsants (sodium valproate).
2 Antituberculous (isoniazid).
3 Cardiovascular drugs (amiodarone; verapamil).
4 Antiulcer drugs (omeprazole; cimetidine).
5 Antibacterials (ciprofloxacin; erythromycin).
6 Antifungals (ketoconazole; fluconazole).
7 Antigout drugs (allopurinol).
8 Sulfonamides.
9 Alcohol (acute intake).

Drugs that affect renal blood supply:
1 NSAIDs.
2 Captopril.
3 Cyclosporine.

Drug-induced renal tubular damage:
1 Aminoglycosides.
2 Thiazides.
3 Lithium.
4 Demeclocycline.
5 Amphotericin B.
6 Cisplatin.

Features of common poisons:
Organophosphorus compounds[1] (pesticides):
1 Constricted pupils.
2 Excessive salivation/sweating.
3 Bradycardia.
4 Bronchospasm (wheezing and rhonchi).
5 Pulmonary oedema (d/t ↑ respiratory secretions) → SOB, frothy sputum and crepitations.
6 NVD.
7 Twitching/convulsions.

Tricyclic antidepressants:[2]
1 Dilated pupils.
2 Dry mouth.
3 Tachycardia; tachyarrhythmias.
4 Bowel sounds absent.
5 Urinary retention.
6 UMN signs.

Barbiturates:
1 Vitals: ↑ PR; ↓ BP; ↓ respiration; ↓ temperature (hypothermia).
2 ↓ conscious level (drowsiness/coma).
3 Bullous skin lesions.

Benzodiazepines:
1 Vitals: ↑ PR; ↓ BP; ↓ respiration.
2 ↓ conscious level (drowsiness/coma).
3 Ataxia.

Salicylates:
1 Hyperventilation.
2 Sweating.
3 Tinnitus; deafness.

Morphine and related alkaloids:
1 Nausea/vomiting – give antiemetic at same time.
2 Hypotension.
3 Respiratory depression.
4 Drowsiness.
5 Pinpoint pupils.
6 Constipation.

---

1 Acetylcholinesterase inhibitors → parasympathomimetic effects.
2 Anticholinergic → parasympatholytic effects.

12 Rheumatology

Muscle pain/stiffness:
1 Normal response to strenuous exercise.
2 Muscle pathology (polymyalgia rheumatica; fibromyalgia).
3 Joint pathology (RA; ankylosing spondylitis).
4 Endocrine pathology (hypothyroidism).
5 Occult malignancy (early manifestation).

Monoarthritis:
1 OA.
2 RA.
3 Infection (tuberculous/pyogenic/gonococcal arthritis).
4 Reactive arthritis (aseptic) – developing about one week after infection elsewhere.
5 Gout/pseudogout.
6 Neuropathic arthritis.
7 Haemarthrosis.
8 Seronegative spondyloarthritides (psoriatic arthritis; Reiter's syndrome).
9 Leukaemic joint deposits.

Polyarthritis:
1 Rheumatoid arthritis.
2 Rheumatic fever.
3 OA.
4 SLE.
5 Seronegative spondyloarthritides (ankylosing spondylitis; enteropathic arthritis; psoriatic arthritis; Reiter's syndrome; Behçet's syndrome).
6 Sjögren's syndrome.
7 Gout.
8 Bacterial infection (gonococcal arthritis).
9 Viral infection (h/o of recent hepatitis A, rubella, mumps or Epstein–Barr viral infection).
10 Drug reaction.

Symmetric polyarthritis:
1 Rheumatoid arthritis (erosive and Rh factor +ve).
2 SLE (non-erosive and ANA +ve).
3 Systemic sclerosis (ANA +ve).
4 Hypogammaglobulinaemia (non-erosive; Rh factor –ve).

Symmetrical periostitis:
1 Hypertrophic pulmonary osteoarthropathy.
2 Vascular insufficiency.
3 Thyroid acropathy.

Extra-articular manifestations of rheumatoid arthritis:
General:
1 Fever.
2 Anorexia; weight loss.
3 Tenosynovitis; bursitis; osteoporosis.
4 Flexion contractures especially of small muscles of hand and feet.
5 Muscular wasting and weakness.
6 Raynaud's phenomenon.
7 Subcutaneous nodules.
8 Lymphadenopathy.

Ocular:
1 Episcleritis; scleritis; scleromalacia.
2 Keratoconjunctivitis sicca (dryness of the eyes).

Pulmonary:
1 Obliterative bronchiolitis.
2 Rheumatoid nodules in the lungs in a patient with pneumoconiosis (Caplan's syndrome).
3 Chronic interstitial fibrosis.
4 Pleurisy.
5 Pleural effusion.

CVS:
1 Cardiomyopathy.
2 Pericarditis.
3 Pericardial effusion.
4 Vasculitis.

Haematological:
1 Anaemia.
2 Thrombocytosis.
3 Felty's syndrome (RA + neutropenia + splenomegaly).

CNS:
1 Cervical cord compression d/t atlanto-axial subluxation.
2 Entrapment neuropathies (carpal tunnel syndrome; tarsal tunnel syndrome [posterior tibial nerve entrapment at ankle joint]; ulnar nerve entrapment at elbow joint).

3 Peripheral neuropathy.

Anaemia in rheumatoid arthritis:
1 Iron-deficiency anaemia (d/t NSAIDs).
2 Folic acid deficiency (d/t ↑ cellular turnover from chronic inflammation).
3 Vitamin B_{12} deficiency (if associated pernicious anaemia present).
4 Anaemia of chronic disease.
5 Hypersplenism (part of Felty's syndrome).
6 Bone marrow suppression (d/t penicillamine; gold).
7 Autoimmune haemolysis.

Eye involvement in rheumatoid arthritis:
1 Episcleritis/scleritis/scleromalacia.
2 Sjögren's syndrome.
3 Cataract (d/t steroid therapy).
4 Retinopathy (d/t chloroquine therapy).
5 Extraocular muscle paralysis (d/t mononeuritis multiplex or penicillamine-induced myasthenia).

Renal involvement in rheumatoid arthritis:
1 NSAIDs induced ATN, acute interstitial nephritis and minimal change GN.
2 Renal papillary necrosis (d/t analgesic abuse).
3 Membranous GN (d/t penicillamine; gold).
4 Amyloidosis.

Pulmonary involvement in rheumatoid arthritis:
1 Larynx (cricoarytenitis).
2 Lungs (pneumonitis; bronchiolitis obliterans; pulmonary nodules; Caplan's syndrome [nodules + progressive massive fibrosis in coal miners]).
3 Pleura (pleural effusion).

Chondrocalcinosis:
1 Gout/pseudogout.
2 OA.
3 Endocrine pathology (hyperparathyroidism; hypothyroidism; hypophosphatasia).
4 Metabolic pathology (haemochromatosis; Wilson's disease).

Pain or limitation of movement in the hand:
1 Recent trauma.
2 Fixed flexion at the ring or little finger:
   a With no palmar fibrosis (trigger finger d/t nodule sticking in tendon sheath).

b With palmar fibrosis (Dupuytren's contracture).
3 RA deformities.
4 Psoriatic arthritis.
5 Lesions around wrist (ganglion; de Quervain's syndrome – stenosing tenosynovitis → wrist pain).
6 Volkmann's ischaemic contracture (flexion deformity at the thumb, fingers, wrist and elbow with forearm pronation).

Dupuytren's contracture:
1 Familial.
2 Alcoholic cirrhosis.
3 Antiepileptic drug therapy.

Pain or limitation of movement at the elbow:
1 Trauma (recent/old).
2 OA.
3 Tennis elbow (epicondylitis).

Pain or limitation of movement at the shoulder:
1 Supraspinatus tendonitis.
2 Rotator cuff tear.
3 Subacromial bursitis.
4 Biceps tendonitis/rupture of long head.
5 Frozen shoulder (adhesive capsulitis).

Pain or limitation of movement at the neck:
1 Torticollis:
  a Infantile torticollis (onset within the first 3 yr).
  b Spasmodic torticollis (d/t recurrent trapezius and sternomastoid spasm) – onset at 10–30 yr.
2 Cervical rib.
3 Anterior/posterior disc prolapse (usually C5/C6 disc prolapse → C6/C7 root compression).

Raynaud's phenomenon:
1 Idiopathic (Raynaud's disease).
2 Vascular causes (thromboangiitis obliterans/Buerger's disease; systemic sclerosis, etc).
3 Cervical causes (cervical rib; cervical spondylosis).
4 Cryoglobulinaemia.
5 Drugs (β-blockers; ergotamine).
6 Trauma (vibrating machine operators).
7 Primary pulmonary hypertension.
8 Occult ca.

Backache:
1 Ligament problem (sprain).
2 Disc problem (herniation).
3 Vertebral problem:
  a Demineralisation (osteoporosis).
  b Inflammation (OA; seronegative spondyloarthritides).
  c Infection (TB – caries spine).
  d Malignancy (multiple myeloma; lymphoma; leukaemia; metastases from ca. prostate, breast, thyroid, etc).
  e Fracture.
4 Pelvic inflammatory disease.

Backache – onset over seconds to hours:
1 Ligament problem (sprain).
2 Disc problem (anterior, posterior or central disc herniation).
3 Vertebral problem (spondylolisthesis).

Backache – onset over days to months:
1 Lumbar spinal stenosis (d/t OA of facet joints).
2 Pyogenic spinal infection of the disc space (by staphylococcus, *Salmonella typhi*, etc).
3 Spinal TB ($\rightarrow$ local abscess $\rightarrow$ cord compression – called Pott's paralysis; psoas abscess).

Backache – onset over years:
1 Kyphotic pain.
2 Scoliotic pain.

Intervertebral disc herniation:
Herniation of the disc b/w L4 and L5 ($\rightarrow$ L5 spinal segment compression):
  ● Weakness of dorsiflexion of the foot; patient unable to walk on heels.
  ● Normal ankle jerk (plantar flexors ok).
  ● Loss of sensation in L5 dermatome (lateral side of leg and dorsum of foot except lateral border).

Herniation of the disc b/w L5 and S1 ($\rightarrow$ S1 spinal segment compression):
  ● Weakness of plantar flexion of the foot; patient unable to walk on toes.
  ● Ankle jerk absent.
  ● Loss of sensation in S1 dermatome (sole including lateral border of the foot and posterior aspect of lower leg).

Spondylolisthesis:
1 Spondylolysis.
2 Congenital malformation of articular process.
3 OA of posterior facet joints.

Osteoporosis:
1 Age (old age; post menopause).
2 Prolonged inactivity d/t any reason (paralysis; stroke, etc).
3 Prolonged steroid therapy.

Sacroiliitis:
1 Seronegative spondyloarthropathies (ankylosing spondylitis; entero-pathic arthritis; psoriatic arthritis; Reiter's syndrome).
2 OA.
3 Whipple's disease.

Spondyloarthropathies – common features:
1 Joints: asymmetrical seronegative (RA factor negative) oligoarthritis; sacroiliitis ($\rightarrow$ hip ache) and/or spondylitis ($\rightarrow$ backache).
2 Tendons: inflammation of tendons – tendonitis.
3 Extra-articular: anterior uveitis.
4 Positive family history.
5 Lab: HLA-B27 – may be positive.

Pain or limitation of movement at the hip:
1 Chronic inflammation (osteoarthritis).
2 Chronic infection (TB).
3 Epiphyseal disease (slipped femoral epiphysis).
4 Perthes' disease.
5 Coxa vara (angle b/w femoral neck and shaft <125°).
6 Developmental dysplasia ($\rightarrow$ dislocation of the hip joint $\rightarrow$ OA).

Avascular necrosis of the femoral head:
1 Local pathology (congenital dislocation of the hip; Perthes' disease; sub-capital fracture of the neck of femur).
2 Systemic pathology (SLE; Cushing's syndrome; sickle-cell anaemia; DM; alcoholism).
3 Iatrogenic (steroid therapy).

Coxa vara (angle b/w femoral neck and shaft <125°):
1 Congenital slipped upper femoral epiphysis.
2 Osteomalacia.
3 Paget's disease.
4 Fracture with malunion or non-union.

Pain or limitation of movement at the knee:
1 Arthritis (acute arthritis [d/t sepsis, RA or gout]; OA).
2 Patellar pathology (chondromalacia patellae; recurrent patellar subluxation; patellar tendinopathy/jumper's knee).
3 Ligamentous injury (meniscal tear/cyst; anterior/posterior cruciate tear; medial/lateral collateral tear; ileotibial tract syndrome).
4 Bursitis with or without infection (e.g. prepatellar bursitis/housemaid's knee, etc).
5 Loose bodies in the knee joint.
6 Medial shelf syndrome (inflamed synovial fold above medial meniscus on arthroscopy).
7 Hoffa's fat syndrome (hypertrophic pad b/w articular surfaces on arthroscopy or MRI).

Loose bodies in the knee joint:
1 Osteophytes in OA.
2 Defective articular surface in osteochondritis dessicans.
3 Chip fractures.
4 Synovial chondromatosis.

Pain or limitation of movement of the foot:
1 Problem with the big toe (hallux valgus; hallux rigidus).
2 Problem with other toes (hammer toes; claw toes).
3 Problem with foot arches (pes planus; pes cavus).
4 Problem with the metatarsals (metatarsalgia; Morton's metatarsalgia d/t interdigital neuroma; march fracture – 2nd or 3rd metatarsal involved).
5 Heel pain (d/t tear of calcaneal tendon; post calcaneal bursitis; arthritis of subtalar joint; plantar fasciitis).

Raised alkaline phosphatase:
1 Paget's disease.
2 Vitamin D deficiency (dietary/$\downarrow$ activation in CRF/resistance).
3 Primary/tertiary hyperparathyroidism.
4 Bone metastases (from thyroid, breast, lungs, kidney, colon and ovary).
5 Obstructive jaundice (cholestasis).

Very high ESR (near or above 100) or CRP:[1]
1 Chronic inflammation (e.g. giant cell arteritis/polymyalgia rheumatica; SLE).
2 Severe bacterial infection (e.g. bacterial endocarditis; empyema; peritonitis; osteomyelitis; sepsis).

---

1 Whereas ESR or CRP levels which are just above the normal are non-specific, an ESR level of near or above 100 is a good lead for certain specific conditions.

3 Malignancy (ca. prostate; myeloma).

Multiple myeloma – diagnostic triad:
1 Plasmacytosis in marrow (>10%).
2 Monoclonal protein band in serum/urine electrophoresis.
3 Evidence of end-organ damage (e.g. lytic bone lesions; hypercalcaemia; renal insufficiency; anaemia).

Differentiation b/w multiple myeloma and monoclonal gammopathy of uncertain significance:[2]
In the latter, we find the following:
1 No urinary Bence–Jones' proteins.
2 Plasmacytosis in marrow (<10%).
3 Monoclonal protein band in serum/urine electrophoresis, but <3 g/dL.
4 No evidence of end-organ damage.

Complications of multiple myeloma:
1 ARF.
2 Amyloidosis.
3 Pathological fractures/cord compression.
4 Recurrent infections.
5 Hyperviscosity syndrome.

Symptoms of hyperviscosity syndrome:
1 Headache.
2 Blurred vision.
3 Vertigo.
4 Coma.

Indications for bone marrow transplantation:
1 Immunodeficiency disorders (e.g. severe combined immunodeficiency).
2 Haemoglobinopathies (e.g. thalassaemia).
3 Aplastic anaemia.
4 Myelophthisic anaemia (multiple myeloma; myelodysplasia; leukaemia; lymphoma).

Antinuclear antibody (ANA):
1 SLE.
2 Sjögren's syndrome.
3 Polymyositis/dermatomyositis.
4 Systemic sclerosis.
5 Rheumatoid arthritis.

---

2   Commoner than multiple myeloma.

Patterns of staining of ANA:
1 Homogeneous:
    a SLE.
2 Speckled:
    a MCTD.
    b Sjögren's syndrome.
3 Nucleolar:
    a Systemic sclerosis.
4 Centromere:
    a CREST syndrome.

Anti-dsDNA antibody:
1 SLE.

Anti-Sm antibody:
1 SLE.
2 Lupoid hepatitis.

Anti-Ro antibody:
1 Sjögren's syndrome.
2 SLE.
3 Congenital neonatal heart block.

Anti-La antibody:
1 Sjögren's syndrome.
2 SLE.

Anti-RNP[3] antibody:
1 MCTD.
2 SLE.

Anti-Jo-1 antibody:
1 Polymyositis.
2 Pulmonary fibrosis.

Anti-Scl-70 antibody:
1 Systemic sclerosis.

---

3   Ribonucleoprotein.

Anti-centromere antibody:
2 CREST syndrome.

Anti-cardiolipin antibody:
1 Antiphospholipid syndrome.
2 SLE.

Anti-histone antibody:
1 Drug-induced SLE.

IgM anti-i antibodies:
1 Mycoplasma pneumonia.[4]

IgG antibodies against the P antigen complex:
1 Paroxysmal nocturnal haemoglobinuria.

cANCA (antigen – proteinase 3 [PR3]):
1 Wegener's granulomatosis.

pANCA (antigen – myeloperoxidase, i.e. anti-MPO subset):
1 Microscopic polyangiitis.
2 Idiopathic crescentic GN.

pANCA (antigens – elastase, lysozyme, lactoferrin):
1 SLE.
2 MCTD.
3 Cryptogenic fibrosing alveolitis (CFA).
4 Ulcerative colitis.
5 Renal tubular acidosis (RTA).
6 Congenital adrenal hyperplasia.

Rheumatoid factor:
1 Connective tissue disorders:
  a Rheumatoid arthritis.
  b Sjögren's syndrome.
  c SLE.
  d Systemic sclerosis.
2 Chronic infections:
  a TB/leprosy.
  b Endocarditis.
3 Others:

---

4 IgM antibodies (cold agglutinins) develop against the I antigen of the erythrocyte membrane.

a Sarcoidosis.
b Lupoid hepatitis.
c Mixed essential cryoglobulinaemia.

Cryoglobulinaemia:[5]
1 Type I (monoclonal Ig):
   a Multiple myeloma.
   b Waldenstrom's macroglobulinaemia.
2 Type II (polyclonal IgG and monoclonal RA factor):
   a Liver pathology (HBV/HCV infection; PBC).
3 Type III (polyclonal IgG and polyclonal RA factor):
   a Hepatitis C.
   b Chronic inflammation (CT disorders – RA; SLE).
   c Lymphoma.

Synovial histology – lymphoid hyperplasia:
1 Rheumatoid arthritis.

Synovial histology – mononuclear cell infiltrate:
1 Hypogammaglobulinaemia.

Positive VDRL test:
1 Syphilis.
2 Antiphospholipid syndrome.

Charcot joint (painless, severely deformed joint):
1 Diabetes mellitus.
2 Syringomyelia.
3 Tabes dorsalis.
4 Leprosy.

PAN – American College of Rheumatology criteria:
1 Weight loss of >4 kg.
2 Testicular pain.
3 Myalgia; leg tenderness.
4 Livedo reticularis.
5 Mono/polyneuropathy.
6 HBsAg positive.
7 Positive biopsy.

---

5 Treatment: plasmapheresis; treatment of the underlying cause; surgery for gangrene, if
   develops.

Duckett Jones' criteria for rheumatic fever:
Jones' major criteria:
1 Migratory arthritis (one or more joints involved).
2 Erythema marginatum (red blotch → fades in the centre and remains red at the edges).
3 Painless subcutaneous nodules.
4 CVS features (pericarditis; systolic murmur; mid-diastolic murmur [Carey Coomb's murmur] d/t nodules over mitral valve; conduction defects; heart failure).

Jones' minor criteria:
1 Arthralgia.
2 ECG: 1st or 2nd degree heart block.
3 Raised ESR.
4 Past h/o rheumatic fever.

Interpretation:
Rheumatic fever = two major criteria, or one major and two minor criteria + evidence of recent streptococcal infection (↑ ASO titre[6] and/or positive throat culture).

Diagnostic criteria for SLE:
(9 clinical; 2 lab)

Clinical:
1 Joints: arthritis – non-erosive; involving >2 joints; deformities uncommon.
2 Malar rash (butterfly rash) – fixed erythema across the nasal bridge and malar eminences.
3 Discoid rash – circular lesions with red, raised margins and scarred, scaly centre; seen over face, neck and other sun-exposed areas.
4 Photosensitivity.
5 Mucous membranes: oral ulcers.
6 CNS: fits; psychosis (without other cause).
7 Cardiopulmonary: pleurisy; pericarditis.
8 Haematological: haemolytic anaemia; leucopenia ($<4 \times 10^9$/L); lymphopenia ($<1.5 \times 10^9$/L); thrombocytopenia ($<100 \times 10^9$/L).
9 Renal: >0.5 g/day proteinuria; 3+ dipstick proteinuria; cellular casts.

Lab:
1 ANF.
2 Anti-dsDNA antibodies; anti-smooth-muscle antibodies; antiphospholipid antibodies.

---

6 Normal ASO titre: in children = up to 330 Todd units; in adults = up to 250 Todd units.

Interpretation:
SLE = 4 or more of the above-mentioned 11 criteria are present.

Diagnostic criteria for Behçet's syndrome:
Major criteria:
1 Recurrent oral ulcers (sine qua non for diagnosis).
2 Genital ulcers.
3 Skin lesions: acne-like lesions; folliculitis; erythema nodosum.
4 Eye: iritis; posterior uveitis; retinal artery/vein occlusion.
5 Pathergy test.[7]

Minor criteria:
1 Intestinal ulcers.
2 Arthritis: non-erosive; most commonly affects ankles/knees.
3 Thrombophlebitis.

Interpretation:
Oral ulceration + at least two of the major criteria are present.

Ankylosing spondylitis – the 'A' disease:
- Arthritis.
- Achilles tendonitis.
- Plantar fasciitis.
- Anterior uveitis.
- Atlanto-axial subluxation.
- Spinal arachnoiditis.
- Apical fibrosis.
- Aortitis/aortic regurgitation.
- AV block.
- IgA nephropathy.
- Amyloidosis.

Polymyositis vs. polymyalgia rheumatica:
1 Muscle tenderness is common in both.
2 Muscle wasting and proximal myopathy is common in polymyositis, but may or may not be present in polymyalgia rheumatica.
3 Headache is usually present in polymyalgia rheumatica; it is absent in polymyositis.
4 In polymyositis alone the following are present:
   a Skin involvement (30%).
   b Raised enzymes (usually).

---

7   A non-specific inflammatory reaction to simple scratching of the skin or following intra-dermal saline injection.

  c Rh factor.
  d ANA (30%).
  e Anti-Jo-1 antibodies (20%).

Diagnostic criteria of adult-onset Still's disease:
Must be present:
1 Quotidian fever >39°C /102°F.
2 Leucocytosis >15 × 10⁹/L.
3 Macular/maculopapular rash.
4 Arthralgia/arthritis.

Plus two of the following:
1 Serositis (pleuritis/pericarditis).
2 Splenomegaly.
3 Generalised lymphadenopathy.
4 Rh factor negative.
5 ANA negative.

Large-vessel vasculitides:
1 Takayasu's arteritis.
2 Temporal arteritis (giant cell arteritis).
3 Behçet's disease (may also involve small/medium sized blood vessels).

Medium-vessel vasculitides:
1 PAN.
2 Buerger's disease.

Small-vessel vasculitides:
Immune-complex mediated:
1 Hypersensitivity vasculitis (cutaneous leucocytoclastic angiitis).
2 Henoch–Schönlein's purpura.
3 Essential cryoglobulinaemia (frequently also involves small/medium sized blood vessels).

ANCA-associated (frequently also involves small/medium-sized blood vessels):
1 Wegener's granulomatosis.
2 Churg–Strauss' syndrome.
3 Microscopic polyangiitis.

Short metacarpals:

1 Turner's syndrome.
2 Noonan's syndrome.
3 Pseudohypoparathyroidism.
4 Sickle-cell dactylitis.
5 Juvenile chronic arthritis.

Rickets and osteomalacia:

1 Vitamin D deficiency (poor intake; malabsorption).
2 Vitamin D-dependent rickets.[8]
3 Renal pathology (CKD; proximal RTA; Fanconi's syndrome).
4 Antiepileptic therapy ($\uparrow$ metabolism of vitamin D to inactive derivatives).
5 Paraneoplastic syndrome.

---

8 Autosomal recessive; two types; in type 1, the defect is $\downarrow$ synthesis of vitamin D; in type 2, the defect is peripheral resistance to vitamin D.

13 Dermatology

Blisters/erosions – immunobullous disorders:
1 Pemphigus vulgaris (PV).
2 Pemphigoid (bullous pemphigoid [BP]; pemphigoid gestationis [PG]; cicatricial pemphigoid [CP]).
3 Dermatitis herpetiformis (DH).

Blisters/erosions – reactive:
1 Toxic epidermal necrolysis (TEN)
2 Staphylococcal scalded skin syndrome (SSSS)
3 Bullous (erythema multiforme [EM]; drug eruptions; insect bites).
4 Acute contact dermatitis (CD).

Blisters/erosions – infections:
1 Herpes (herpes simplex; herpes zoster [shingles]; varicella zoster [chicken pox]).
2 Bullous impetigo.
3 Cellulitis (occasionally, if severe).

Blisters/erosions – miscellaneous:
1 Porphyria (cutanea tarda and variegata).
2 Pompholyx (dyshidrotic eczema).
3 Diabetic bullae.
4 Burns.

Blisters/erosions in a middle/old-age patient:
1 PV.
2 Pemphigoid (BP; CP).
3 PCT (porphyria cutanea tarda).

Blisters/erosions in a child/young adult:
1 Pemphigoid (PG).
2 DH.
3 Chicken pox.
4 Bullous impetigo (exclusively in children).
5 SSSS (exclusively in children).

Blisters/erosions – duration:
1 Short history (hours/days): 'reactive' causes, and 'infections'.

2 Long history (weeks/months): immunobullous disorders and porphyria.

Blisters/erosions – painful:
1 Herpes (herpes zoster and eczema herpeticum).
2 Cellulitis.
3 TEN.
4 SSSS.
5 Widespread erosions are painful, regardless of the cause, especially if secondarily infected.

Blisters/erosions – itching:
1 DH.
2 Pemphigoid (BP; PG).
3 Pompholyx.
4 Chicken pox.
5 Contact dermatitis.
6 Insect bites.

Blisters/erosions – positive drug history:
1 EM.
2 TEN.
3 Bullous drug eruptions.

Blisters/erosions – pregnancy:
1 PG.

Blisters/erosions – suggestive occupational history:
1 Contact dermatitis.[1]

Blisters/erosions– sites – mucous membranes:
1 PV.
2 Pemphigoid (CP).
3 EM and TEN (lips affected too).

Blisters/erosions – sites – centripetal:
1 Chicken pox.
2 Pemphigoid (PG – often begins on the abdomen).

Blisters/erosions – sites – limbs:
1 DH (extensor surfaces, especially knees and elbows).
2 EM (particularly hands and feet).
3 Pompholyx (palms, soles and sides of digits).

---

1 Gardener with rash on the hands: CD d/t allergy to a plant.

4 Diabetic bullae (lower legs).

5 Insect bites ('clustered' lesions anywhere along the limbs).

Blisters/erosions – sites – dermatomal:

1 Herpes zoster.

Blisters/erosions – sites – photosensitive (distribution over light-exposed areas):

1 Porphyrias (cutanea tarda[2] and variegata).

2 Photosensitive drug eruptions.

Blisters/erosions – sites – localised and asymmetric:

1 Infections (herpes simplex [often clustered]; bullous impetigo; cellulitis).

2 CD.

Positive Nikolsky's sign:[3]

1 PV.

2 TEN.

3 SSSS.

Chronic red facial rash – common causes:

1 Dermatitis (atopic dermatitis; seborrhoeic dermatitis; contact dermatitis).

2 Acne.

3 Rosacea.

4 Tinea faciei.

Chronic red facial rash – less common causes:

1 LE (SLE; DLE).

2 Dermatomyositis.

3 Sarcoidosis.

4 Photosensitive eczema (endogenous and exogenous).

Erythroderma – endogenous causes:

1 Psoriasis (pustular and non-pustular).

2 Eczema.

3 Sézary's syndrome.

4 Pityriasis rubra pilaris (PRP).

5 Paraneoplastic.

---

2 Associated with liver problems like hepatitis C or alcoholic liver disease.

3 If shearing force is applied to apparently normal perilesional skin, there occurs epidermal detachment.

Erythroderma – 'reactive':
1 Drug eruptions.
2 Allergic contact dermatitis.
3 TEN.
4 Infectious exanthemata (TSS; SSSS).

Pruritus without a rash:
1 Obstructive liver disease.
2 CRF.
3 Iron-deficiency anaemia.
4 Polycythaemia rubra vera.
5 Haemolytic malignancy (especially lymphoma).
6 Hyper- and hypothyroidism.
7 Dry skin.
8 Drugs.
9 Psychological.

Pruritus with a rash:
1 Eczema.
2 Lichen planus.
3 Urticaria.
4 Scabies and other infestations.
5 Dermatitis herpetiformis.
6 Bullous pemphigoid.
7 Pityriasis rosea.
8 Sézary's syndrome.
9 Insect bite.
10 Drug eruptions.

Telogen effluvium:
1 Parturition and abortion.
2 Major surgery.
3 Major illness.
4 Fever.
5 Drugs.
6 Emotional stress.
7 Crash dieting.

Anagen effluvium:
1 Cytotoxic drugs.
2 Poisoning (e.g. heavy metals).

Alopecia – scarring (often patchy):
1 DLE.

2 Lichen planus (LP).
3 Cicatricial pemphigoid (CP).
4 Sarcoidosis.
5 Infections (including fungal kerion)
6 Tumours (e.g. basal cell carcinoma).
7 Radiation/burns.
8 Traction (late stages).

Alopecia – non-scarring and patchy:
1 Androgenic alopecia.
2 Alopecia areata.
3 Tinea capitis.
4 Secondary syphilis.
5 Traction (late stages).

Alopecia – non-scarring and generalised:
1 Telogen/anagen effluvium.
2 Alopecia totalis.
3 Iron-deficiency anaemia.
4 SLE.
5 Malnutrition.
6 Endocrine (e.g. thyroid disease; hypopituitarism).
7 Any chronic disease.
8 Drugs.

Patch/plaque on the lower leg – tumours:
1 Basal/squamous cell ca.
2 Malignant melanoma.
3 Kaposi's sarcoma.
4 Bowen's disease.

Patch/plaque on the lower leg – inflammatory conditions:
1 Eczema (discoid; venous).
2 Hypertrophic lichen planus.

Patch/plaque on the lower leg – infections:
1 Cellulitis.
2 Tinea.
3 Erythema chronicum migrans (Lyme disease).

Patch/plaque on the lower leg – endocrine causes:
1 Pretibial myxoedema.
2 Necrobiosis lipoidica.

Patch/plaque on the lower leg – miscellaneous:
1 Erythema nodosum.
2 Morphoea.
3 Granuloma annulare.

Leg ulcerations – tumours:
1 Basal/squamous cell ca.
2 Malignant melanoma.
3 Kaposi's sarcoma.

Leg ulcerations – vasculitis:
Large-vessel disease:
1 Venous ulceration.
2 Atherosclerosis.
3 Polyarteritis nodosa.
4 Systemic sclerosis.

Small-vessel disease:
1 Diabetes mellitus.
2 Connective tissue disorders (RA; SLE; systemic sclerosis; cutaneous vasculitis).

Leg ulcerations – blood abnormalities:
1 Sickle-cell anaemia.
2 Cryoglobulinaemia.
3 Immune-complex disease.

Leg ulcerations – neuropathy:
1 Diabetes mellitus.
2 Leprosy.
3 Syphilis.

Leg ulcerations – infections:
1 Mycobacterium.
2 Fungal.
3 Pyoderma gangrenosum.

Leg ulcerations – miscellaneous:
1 Trauma.
2 Necrobiosis lipoidica.

Abnormal skin pigmentation – genetic conditions:
1 Albinism.
2 Neurofibromatosis ($\rightarrow$ café au lait spots).

3 Tuberous sclerosis ($\rightarrow$ ash-leaf spots).

Neurofibromatosis – associated peripheral abnormalities:
1 Renal artery stenosis.
2 Phaeochromocytoma.
3 Cardiomyopathy (hypertrophic; dilated; restrictive).
4 Pulmonary fibrosis.
5 Fibrous dysplasia of bone.

Neurofibromatosis – associated central abnormalities:
1 Acoustic neuroma.
2 Optic glioma.
3 Meningioma.
4 Ependymoma.

Hypopigmentation – localised:
1 Vitiligo.
2 Halo naevi.
3 Pityriasis versicolor.
4 Postinflammatory hypopigmentation.
5 Leprosy.
6 Chemicals (therapeutic/occupational use of hydroquinone, p-tertiary butyl phenol).

Hypopigmentation – generalised:
1 Generalised vitiligo (islands of normal skin also present).
2 Hypopituitarism (d/t lack of MSH).

Hyperpigmentation – localised:
1 Freckles.
2 Melasma.
3 Acanthosis nigricans.
4 Postinflammatory hyperpigmentation.
5 Haemosiderosis.
6 Alkaptonuria (ochronosis).
7 Drugs (minocycline; chlorpromazine; amiodarone; DMARDs – chloroquine, gold).

Hyperpigmentation – generalised:
1 Addison's disease; Nelson's syndrome.
2 Ectopic ACTH/MSH (lung ca.; carcinoid tumour).
3 Addison's-like hyperpigmentation in other endocrinopathies (phaeochromocytoma; Cushing's syndrome; acromegaly; hyperthyroidism).
4 GI (malnutrition; malabsorption).

5 Liver (hyperbilirubinaemia; hypercarotenaemia; cirrhosis d/t any cause especially haemochromatosis and PBC).
6 CRF.
7 Systemic sclerosis.
8 Drugs (cytotoxic drugs – busulfan; bleomycin; cyclophosphamide; mepacrine).

Pigmentation of the previously non-pigmented scars:
1 Melanosis.
2 Addison's disease.

Erythema nodosum:
1 Chronic inflammation: sarcoidosis; IBD; Behçet's syndrome.
2 Infections: bacterial (streptococci; AFB: yersinia); viral (EBV); fungal (coccidioidomycosis; trichophyton).
3 Malignancy (e.g. lymphoma).
4 Drugs (sulfonamides; OCPs).

Diseases associated with pyoderma gangrenosum:
1 Idiopathic (50%).
2 GI: IBD.
3 Liver: chronic active hepatitis; PBC; sclerosing cholangitis.
4 Joints: RA; seronegative arthropathies.
5 Vasculitides (Wegener's granulomatosis).
6 Malignancy: myeloma (paraproteinaemia); ca. colon, prostate, breast; leukaemia/lymphoma.
7 Endocrine diseases: DM; thyroid disease.
8 At sites of trauma (Koebner's phenomenon).

Carotenaemia:
1 ↑ intake of carotene (overeating mangoes, carrots – 4kg/day).
2 Myxoedema (→ ↓ enzymatic conversion of carotene to vitamin A).
3 Hyperbetalipoproteinaemia.

Genital papule/ulcer with inguinal lymphadenopathy:
1 Syphilis (painless; d/t *Treponema pallidum*).
2 Chancroid (painful; d/t *Haemophilus ducreyi*).
3 Lymphogranuloma venereum (d/t *Chlamydia trachomatis*).
4 Granuloma inguinale (d/t *Klebsiella granulomatis*; appears as Donovan bodies on gram staining).

Acanthosis nigricans:
1 Occult malignancy (ca. stomach/lung; lymphoma).
2 Diabetes mellitus.

3 As an isolated abnormality.

Yellow-nail syndrome:
1 Chronic lung disease.
2 Peripheral lymphoedema.

Koebner's phenomenon:
1 Psoriasis.
2 Lichen planus.
3 Vitiligo.
4 Bullous pemphigoid.
5 Molluscum contagiosum.
6 Viral warts.

Orogenital ulceration:
1 Seronegative spondyloarthropathies (Behçet's syndrome; Reiter's syndrome).
2 IBD (Crohn's disease; ulcerative colitis).
3 Skin pathologies (lichen planus; EM; SJS; TEN).
4 Infections (HCV; HIV; HSV; syphilis; gonococcal infection).

Orogenital ulceration and venous thromboses:
1 Seronegative spondyloarthropathies (Behçet's syndrome; Reiter's syndrome).
2 IBD (Crohn's disease; ulcerative colitis).

Livedo reticularis:
1 Physiological.
2 Vasculitis.
3 Hyperviscosity syndrome/thrombocythaemia.
4 Cryoglobulinaemia.
5 Cholesterol emboli.
6 Heart failure.
7 Paralysis.
8 Drug-induced (amantadine).

Cutaneous manifestations of ca. lung:
1 Dermatomyositis.
2 Acanthosis palmaris.
3 Erythema gyratum repens.

Cutaneous manifestations of lymphoma:
1 Hypertrichosis (Hodgkin's lymphoma).
2 Ichthyosis.

3 Pyoderma gangrenosum (lymphoma; leukaemia).

A continuous band of IgM and C_3b at dermoepidermal junction:

1 SLE (the band is called 'lupus band').

14 Ophthalmology

Angioid streaks:
1 Pituitary disorder (acromegaly etc).
2 Bone disorder (Paget's disease).
3 Connective tissue disorder (Ehlers–Danlos' syndrome; pseudoxanthoma elasticum).
4 Blood disorder (sickle-cell disease).

Band keratopathy:
1 Chronic uveitis.
2 Hypercalcaemia.

Bitot's spots:
1 Vitamin A deficiency.

Black sunburst (chorioretinal scar):
1 Sickle-cell disease.

Blue sclera:
1 Osteogenesis imperfecta (blue sclera + multiple/recurrent fractures d/t bone fragility).
2 Osteosclerosis (blue sclera + deafness).
3 Marfan's syndrome.
4 Ehlers–Danlos' syndrome.
5 Pseudoxanthoma elasticum.
6 Hyperthyroidism.

Brushfield's spots:
1 Down's syndrome.

Kayser–Fleischer's ring:
1 Wilson's disease.

Lisch's nodules:
1 Neurofibromatosis.

Heterochromia of the iris:
1 Normal with no clinical significance.
2 Wearing contact lenses of different colours.

Sudden loss of vision:
1 Vascular problem:
   a Vascular occlusion (temporal arteritis; central retinal artery/vein occlusion).
   b Haemorrhage (vitreous haemorrhage).
2 Neuronal problem:
   a Nerve problem (optic and retrobulbar neuritis; ischaemic optic neuropathy).
   b Visual field problem (homonymous hemianopia).
3 Problem with the eyeball layers (retinal detachment; choroiditis).

Gradual loss of vision:
1 Refractive errors (myopia; hypermetropia; presbyopia).
2 Cataract.
3 Glaucoma.
4 Problem with the eyeball layers (diabetic retinopathy; retinitis pigmentosa; macular degeneration; chorioretinitis; malignant melanoma of the choroid).
5 Nerve problem (tumour of the optic nerve [glioma or meningioma]; optic chiasmal disease, e.g. compression d/t pituitary tumour or meningioma; vitamin B deficiency amblyopia).

Transient loss of vision (for a few minutes or hours):
1 Migraine.
2 Temporary vascular occlusion d/t retinal emboli from internal carotid artery – known as amaurosis fugax.
3 Giant cell ('temporal') arteritis: can cause transient loss of vision but more likely to cause permanent severe loss, often bilaterally.[1]
4 Papilloedema (d/t SOL brain, malignant hypertension, benign intracranial hypertension etc).[2]
5 Subacute glaucoma (several attacks of subacute glaucoma may precede an attack of acute closed-angle glaucoma).

Blindness in the developed world:
1 Patient >65 years of age: commonest cause = macular degeneration.
2 Young patient: commonest cause = diabetic retinopathy.
3 Glaucoma.
4 Trauma.
5 Congenital.

---

1 Emboli cannot reach the retina from the temporal artery, and loss of vision in temporal arteritis is not the result of embolism but rather d/t occlusion of the posterior cilliary vesels by intimal vessel-wall thickening.

2 Papilloedema → vascular occlusion within the optic nerve.

Blindness in the developing world:
1 Infections (trachoma caused by *Chlamydia trachomatis*; onchocerciasis caused by a parasite, *Onchocerca volvulus* [known as river blindness]).
2 Nutritional deficiency like xerophthalmia caused by vitamin A deficiency.
3 Cataract.
4 Chronic glaucoma.

Acute red eye:
1 Inflammation of the anterior part of the eye (conjunctivitis; keratitis; episcleritis; scleritis; uveitis).
2 Subconjunctival haemorrhage.
3 Acute closed-angle glaucoma – emergency.

Conjunctivitis:
1 Bacterial infection (*S. aureus*; *S. pyogenes*; *H. influenzae*; coliforms).
2 Chlamydial infection (although a bacteria, it produces two distinct ocular entities – trachoma (chronic form of the disease) and inclusion conjunctivitis (acute form of the disease).
3 Viral infection (adenovirus).
4 Allergic (e.g. to pollens [hay fever] or eye drops).

Keratitis:
1 Bacterial (*S. aureus*; *S. pneumoniae*; pseudomonas; enterobacteria).
2 Viral (herpes simplex virus; herpes zoster virus).
3 Fungal (*Candida albicans*; aspergillus).
4 Non-infective (secondary to wearing hard contact lenses or exposure to high doses of UV light).

Corneal ulcer (ulcerative keratitis):
1 Abrasion.
2 Infection (herpes simplex; pseudomonas; candida; aspergillus; protozoa).

Corneal arcus:
1 Physiologic (in old age).
2 Hypercholesterolaemia.

Corneal calcification:
1 Chronic renal failure.
2 Hypercalcaemia (d/t hyperparathyroidism, vitamin D intoxication, sarcoidosis, etc).

Acute iritis (anterior uveitis) – circumcorneal injection:
1 Idiopathic in most cases.
2 Trauma (usually surgery).

3 Infection (herpes simplex; herpes zoster; TB; leprosy; syphilis; fungal; protozoal).
4 Autoimmune diseases like seronegative spondyloarthritides (i.e. ankylosing spondylitis, enteropathic arthritis; Reiter's syndrome and Behçet's syndrome); chronic juvenile arthritis; immune ocular disease.
5 Sarcoidosis.

Chronic iritis:
1 Chronic inflammation:
   a Juvenile rheumatoid arthritis (Still's disease).
2 Chronic infection:
   a TB.
   b Leprosy.

Episcleritis:
1 Idiopathic in most cases.
2 Rheumatoid arthritis.

Scleritis:
1 Commonest cause = rheumatoid arthritis.
2 Connective tissue disorders (e.g. Wegener's granulomatosis; polyarteritis nodosa).
3 Gout.

Subconjunctival haemorrhage:
1 Spontaneous (especially in middle- and old-age people).
2 Trauma.

Irritable eye (itching, burning or sore eye):
Eyelid problem:
1 Inflammation of the eyelid margin (called blepharitis) usually d/t chronic staphylococcal infection.
2 In-turning lashes (d/t entropion or trichiasis).
3 Poor lid closure (d/t facial palsy or severe proptosis) leading to dryness of the eye.

Conjunctival problem:
1 Chronic allergic conjunctivitis.
2 Chronic viral conjunctivitis (d/t papovavirus or molluscum virus).

Dry eye:
Lacrimal gland is diseased:
1 ↓ lacrimal gland secretion (called keratoconjunctivitis sicca) d/t rheumatoid arthritis, Sjögren's syndrome, sarcoidosis, etc.

Conjunctiva is diseased (scarred) d/t:

1 Conjunctival inflammation d/t unknown aetiology (ocular pemphigoid).
2 Infection (trachoma).
3 Thermal/chemical injury.
4 Nutritional deficiency (vitamin A deficiency).

Watering of the eye:

↑ Formation of the tears (lacrimation):

1 Foreign body.
2 In-turning lashes (d/t entropion or trichiasis).

↓ Drainage of the tears (epiphora):

1 Lower lid is displaced (ectropion [lid turns outwards] and facial palsy [lid falls away from the eyeball] so that tears collect and then spill from the lower conjunctival sac).
2 Canaliculi are obstructed (caused by chronic infection with staph. or streptothrix, or trauma).
3 Stenosis of the nasolacrimal duct.

Unilateral ptosis:

Congenital:

1 Congenital weakness of the levator muscle.

Acquired:

1 Idiopathic
2 Neurogenic (3rd nerve palsy; Horner's syndrome).
3 Myogenic (senile degeneration of the levator muscle; myasthenia gravis; dystrophia myotonica).
4 Mechanical (swelling of the upper eye lid d/t inflammation, tumour or some vascular abnormality).

Bilateral ptosis:

1 Neurogenic (bilateral Horner's syndrome [syringomyelia]; tabes dorsalis).
2 Myogenic (senile degeneration of the levator muscle; myasthenia gravis; dystrophia myotonica; ocular myopathy; mitochondrial dystrophy).

Lid retraction:

1 Graves' disease (also called thyroid ophthalmopathy). The mechanism is probably sympathetic overactivity of the Müller's muscle.

Entropion:

1 Senile.
2 Cicatricial (d/t trachoma or trauma → inflammation → fibrosis → entropion).

Ectropion:
1 Senile.
2 Cicatricial (d/t trauma, or tumour arising from the eyelid skin).

Trichiasis:
1 Scarring of the eyelid margin (secondary to infection or trauma).

Blepharitis (inflammation of the eyelid margin):
1 Infection (usually staphylococcal).

Stye (inflammation of the lash follicle):
1 Infection (usually staphylococcal).

Dacryoadenitis (inflammation of the lacrimal gland):
1 Viral infection, e.g. mumps.
2 Sarcoidosis.

Proptosis (forward protrusion of the eye + lids):
1 Ophthalmic Graves' disease ± thyrotoxicosis (commonest cause of both unilateral and bilateral proptosis).
2 Orbital cellulitis (usually an extension from frontal or ethmoidal sinusitis). It is a medical emergency.
3 Orbital tumour (rarely primary; often secondary, especially reticulosis).
4 Orbital haematoma (usually secondary to head injury).
5 Vascular problem (caroticocavernous fistula).

Dilated pupil (mydriasis):
Unilateral:
1 3rd nerve palsy (unilateral mydriasis + light and accommodation reflexes absent).
2 Traumatic iridoplegia (h/o direct trauma + fixed, dilated, irregular pupil that neither accommodates nor reacts to light; confirmed by slit lamp examination of the anterior chamber).
3 Holmes–Adie's pupil (d/t ciliary ganglion degeneration).
4 Mydriatic eye drops – unilateral.

Bilateral:
1 Mydriatic eye drops (atropine) – bilateral.
2 Drugs (anticholinergics; tricyclics; cocaine; amphetamines; poisoning with CO or ethylene glycol).
3 Midbrain damage.

Constricted pupil (miosis):
Unilateral:
1 Horner's syndrome (unilateral miosis + light and accommodation reflexes present).
2 Miotic eye drops – unilateral.

Bilateral:
1 Miotic eye drops (pilocarpine) – bilateral.
2 Drugs (narcotic/barbiturate overdose; organophosphorus poisoning).
3 Pontine lesion.
4 Argyll Robertson's pupils (bilateral miosis + pupillary reflex absent + accommodation reflex present).
5 Age-related miosis (d/t autonomic degeneration).

Pupillary reactions in the unconscious patient:
Unilateral dilated non-reacting pupil:
1 Ipsilateral 3rd nerve involvement (d/t brainstem compression or herniation of the cerebral hemispheres through the tentorium).

Bilateral dilated non-reacting pupils:
1 Bilateral 3rd nerve involvement: ditto.

Bilateral constricted pupils:
1 Pontine lesion.

Pupillary size and reaction to light:
1 Dilated (≥6 mm) not reacting to light:
   a Midbrain lesion.
   b 3rd nerve palsy.
2 Mid-position (3–5 mm):
   a Reacting to light:
      i Excludes midbrain lesion.
   b Not reacting to light:
      i Lesion is at midbrain–pons junction.
3 Small pupil (1–3 mm) reacting to light:
   a Lesion is above brainstem.
   b Metabolic encephalopathy.
4 Small pinpoint (<1 mm) pupil reacting to light:
   a Pontine haemorrhage.
   b Narcotic overdose.

White pupil (leucocoria):
Lens is diseased:
1 Cataract.

Retina is diseased:
1 Retinoblastoma.
2 Retinopathy of prematurity.

Monocular diplopia (double vision persists even after covering one eye):
1 Corneal scarring.
2 Astigmatism.
3 Cataract.

Binocular diplopia (double vision disappears on covering one eye):
Neurogenic:
1 3rd, 4th or 6th nerve palsy, or ischaemic of the motor nuclei of these nerves in the brainstem (d/t occlusion of the vertebrobasilar artery).

Myogenic:
1 Myasthenia gravis (diplopia + ptosis + dysphagia).
2 Graves' disease (thyroid ophthalmopathy).

Mechanical:
1 Displacement of the eyeball (by an orbital tumour or a 'blow-out' fracture of the orbital floor).

Lens dislocation:
1 Trauma.
2 Uveal tumour.
3 Refsum's disease.[3]
4 Homocystinuria (downwards).[4]
5 Marfan's syndrome (upwards).[5]
6 Ehlers–Danlos' syndrome.[6]
7 Weill–Marchesani's syndrome.[7]

Papilloedema:
With sudden loss of vision:
1 Central retinal vein occlusion; optic neuritis; ischaemic optic neuropathy.

---

3 Ectopia lentis, retinitis pigmentosa, cerebellar ataxia and polyneuropathy.
4 Fair skin, coarse hair, mental retardation (learning difficulties), seizures, ectopia lentis, osteoporosis and thromboembolism.
5 Tall, lean, long extremities, long fingers/toes, flat feet, stooped shoulders, abnormal joint flexibility, ectopia lentis and aortic aneurysm.
6 Hyperelasticity of skin and joints, poor wound healing, ectopia lentis, aortic aneurysm/dissection and medullary sponge kidney.
7 Short stature, skeletal abnormalities and ectopia lentis.

Intact vision:
1 ↑ ICP (d/t a SOL [e.g. haematoma, abscess, cyst, tumour]; meningitis; encephalitis; CVA, e.g. SAH).
2 Venous obstruction (e.g. cavernous sinus thrombosis).
3 HTN (malignant/accelerated/benign intracranial HTN).
4 'Severe' hypoxia, hypercapnia or anaemia.

Optic atrophy:
Retinal disease:
1 Central retinal artery occlusion; retinitis pigmentosa.

Optic nerve disease:
1 Chronic glaucoma (commonest cause of optic atrophy).
2 Optic (retrobulbar) neuritis.
3 Ischaemic optic neuropathy.

Optic chiasmal disease:
1 Compression of the optic chiasma (d/t pituitary tumour, etc).

Horner's syndrome:
Lesion is within the CNS:
1 SOL (→ exogenous compression); ischaemia (d/t thrombosis of the posterior inferior cerebellar artery); demyelination (d/t multiple sclerosis).

Lesion is outside the CNS between thoracic outlet and superior cervical ganglion:
1 Pancoast's tumour.
2 Thyroid swelling.
3 Cervical rib.

Lesion is outside the CNS distal to the superior cervical ganglion:
1 Iatrogenic (during surgical exploration of the neck or carotid arteriography).

Eye movements:
Unconscious patient:
1 Doll's-eye movements positive: brainstem intact; cerebral hemispheres damaged.
2 Doll's-eye movements absent: brainstem lesion.

Conjugate eye movements:
1 Cerebral hemisphere pathology: eyes deviate towards the side of the lesion.
2 Brainstem pathology: eyes deviate away from the side of the lesion.

Roth's spots:
1 Inflammatory causes (infective endocarditis; SLE; PAN).
2 Severe anaemia.
3 Malignancy (leukaemia).

Advanced diabetic eye disease:
- Vitreous haemorrhage.
- Retinal detachment.
- Rubeotic glaucoma.

Diabetic maculopathy:
1 Loss of central vision (peripheral vision spared).
2 Macular oedema + macular stars (hard exudates arranged in a horseshoe or circular fashion around the macula).

Diabetic retinopathy – criteria for referral to an ophthalmologist:
1 Preproliferative/proliferative retinopathy.
2 Maculopathy.
3 Advanced diabetic eye disease.

Cotton-wool spots:
1 Diabetes mellitus.
2 Hypertension.
3 Septicaemia.
4 Vasculitis.
5 HIV retinopathy.
6 Myeloproliferative disorders.

Retinal vein thrombosis:
1 Diabetes mellitus.
2 Hypertension.
3 Glaucoma.
4 Hyperviscosity (polycythaemia; myeloma; macroglobulinaemia).
5 Vasculitides.

Retinal artery occlusion:
1 Thrombosis.
2 Embolism (AF; carotid artery stenosis).
3 Vasculitides (especially giant cell arteritis).
4 Exogenous compression (d/t ↑ intraorbital pressure).
5 Spasm (cocaine; retinal migraine).
6 Sickle-cell disease.
7 Syphilis.

Retinitis pigmentosa:

1 Familial (autosomal dominant, recessive, X-linked).
2 Friedreich's ataxia.
3 Refsum's disease.
4 Abetalipoproteinaemia.
5 Laurence–Moon–Biedl's syndrome.
6 Bassen–Kornzweig's syndrome (retinitis pigmentosa + abetalipo-proteinaemia).
7 Kearns–Sayre's syndrome.[8]

---

8 Retinitis pigmentosa, optic atrophy, mitochondrial myopathy with muscle biopsy showing red-ragged fibres.

15 Psychiatry

Collapsed patient in a psychiatry ward:
1 Neuroleptic malignant syndrome.
2 Epilepsy (d/t neuroleptic agents or psychogenic polydipsia [$\rightarrow \downarrow Na^+$]).
3 Torsades de pointes (d/t neuroleptic agents, lithium or TCA overdose).
4 Sedative overdose.
5 Diabetic emergencies (d/t olanzapine).

Unconscious alcoholic:
1 Alcohol intoxication; methanol poisoning; ethylene glycol poisoning.
2 Encephalopathy (hepatic; Wernicke's).
3 Meningitis (tuberculous).
4 Haemorrhage (SAH; variceal/peptic ulcer bleed; acute haemorrhagic pancreatitis).
5 Alcohol-induced hypoglycaemia.

Anxiety disorders – clinical features:
1 CNS: anxious thoughts; headache.
2 Respiratory system: SOB/hyperventilation.
3 CVS: palpitations; chest pain.
4 GIT: nausea; loose motions.
5 UT: $\uparrow$ urinary frequency.
6 Limbs: tingling.

Anxiety states:
1 Psychogenic (commonest cause) – generalised anxiety disorder; panic disorder.
2 Hyperthyroidism (common).
3 Tachyarrhythmia (e.g. SVT – fairly common).
4 Alcohol withdrawal (h/o excessive alcohol intake).
5 Hypoglycaemia.
6 Phaeochromocytoma (rare).

Anxiety in response to specific issues:
1 Eating disorder (anorexia nervosa; bulimia nervosa).
2 Somatisation disorder (Briquet's syndrome).
3 Phobias (social phobia; agoraphobia [crowd phobia or situations where escape is difficult]; claustrophobia [fear of enclosed spaces]; arachnophobia [fear of spiders]).

4 Post-traumatic stress disorders (caused by experiencing or witnessing a traumatic event, e.g. major accident, fire, assault, military combat).

Depression – clinical features:
1 Worse in the evening (diurnal variation).
2 Anhedonia.[1]
3 Loss of concentration, retardation.
4 Decreased libido, sleep disorder (early-morning awakening), loss of appetite, weight loss.

Bipolar affective disorder – clinical features:
1 Symptoms are mainly of increased mood:
2 Elevated mood.
3 Flight of ideas, pressure of speech, delusions of grandeur, poor attention span.
4 Insomnia, loss of inhibition, increased libido, increased appetite but weight loss.

Depression – causes:
1 Depression (mild to moderate; major).
2 Depression secondary to other conditions (anxiety disorder; alcohol/substance abuse).
3 Depression secondary to medication (β-blockers; α-blockers; Ca^{2+} channel blockers; corticosteroids; OCPs; antipsychotics; antiparkinsonism [levodopa]).
4 Seasonal affective disorder.

Hallucinations, delusions or thought disorders:[2]
1 Mania or hypomania.
2 Bipolar disorder.
3 Acute/chronic schizophrenia.

Acute delirium (confusional state):
1 Infection (CNS infection, i.e. meningitis, encephalitis; septicaemia; UTI; pneumonia).
2 Hypoxia.
3 Intracerebral pathology, e.g. head injury, haemorrhage or tumour.
4 Metabolic disturbance, e.g. uraemic/hepatic encephalopathy, hypoglycaemia, hypercalcaemia.
5 Endocrinopathy (hyper- or hypothyroidism; DM; Cushing's).
6 Drugs (especially in elderly).

---

1 Loss of pleasure from acts which ordinarily would be pleasurable.
2 Thoughts jump from one idea to another in a bizarre way.

7 Alcohol (acute intoxication/withdrawal syndrome).

Chronic confusion:
1 Alzheimer's dementia (dementia in the absence of cerebral infarction/ parkinsonism).
2 Vascular (multi-infarct) dementia (progression of dementia with each subsequent infarct).
3 Lewy-body dementia (dementia with parkinsonism and hallucinations).
4 Other neurodegenerative diseases (Huntington's chorea; bovine spongi-form encephalopathy).

Schizophrenia – first-rank symptoms:
1 Auditory hallucinations:
  a Third-person voices discussing the patient.
  b Audible thoughts/echoes.
  c Commentary on actions.
2 Passivity:
  d Thought insertion, withdrawal or broadcast.
  e Feeling of thoughts/actions being under external control.
3 Delusions.

Eating disorders (anorexia/bulimia nervosa) – complications:
1 Vitals: dehydration → hypotension, hypokalaemia; hypothermia.
2 Brain: reversible brain atrophy; seizures.
3 CVS: arrhythmias; bradycardia.
4 Lipid profile: hypercholesterolaemia.
5 GIT: dental erosions/decay; GI erosions/ulcerations.
6 Kidneys: nephropathy.
7 Endocrinopathy: ↓ FSH/LH → ↓ oestrogen → amenorrhoea.
8 Bone: osteoporosis (→ ↑ risk of fractures).
9 Bone marrow: hypoplastic bone marrow (→ pancytopenia).
10 Muscles: proximal myopathy; cramps; tetany.

Obsessive compulsive disorder – associations:
1 Anorexia nervosa.
2 Schizophrenia.
3 Organic brain disease.

Suicide – risk factors:
1 Gender: male.
2 Age: young or late middle age.
3 Social history: social class I or V; alcoholic; unemployed.
4 H/o: chronic illness/ pain; physically handicap; psychiatric problem.

Acute alcohol withdrawal (delirium tremens) – clinical features:
Onset after 72 hours without alcohol.

1 Tremors; pyrexia.
2 Visual hallucinations.
3 Confused; agitated; insomnia.
4 Look for: associated infection, electrolyte abnormalities (K$^+$; Mg^{2+}).

Wernicke's encephalopathy[3] – clinical features:

1 Confused.
2 Gait: ataxia.
3 Eyes: nystagmus; abducens and conjugate gaze palsies; ophthalmoplegia.
4 Limbs: peripheral neuropathy.

Wernicke's encephalopathy – causes:

1 Alcoholism.
2 Dietary deficiency; malabsorption; repeated persistent vomiting (d/t any cause).
3 Pregnancy ($\uparrow$ demand; hyperemesis gravidarum).
4 Dialysis.

Korsakoff's syndrome – clinical features:

1 Memory: markedly impaired short-term recall despite normal registration; anterograde amnesia; variable retrograde amnesia.
2 Confabulation.
3 Lack of insight.

Korsakoff's syndrome – causes:

1 Wernicke's encephalopathy.
2 Herpes simplex encephalopathy.
3 CO poisoning.

Electroconvulsive therapy (ECT) – contraindications:

1 $\uparrow$ ICP (absolute).
2 Brain tumour (relative).
3 Cardiac arrhythmia.
4 Recent MI/CVA.

Electroconvulsive therapy (ECT) – side effects:

1 Fractures/dislocations.
2 Headache; confusion; $\downarrow$ short-term memory.

---

3   Caused by acute thiamine deficiency.

16 Ear, nose and throat (ENT)

External ear abnormalities:
1 Congenital anomalies.
2 Infected preauricular sinus.
3 Painful nodules on the upper margin of the pinna in men (chondroder-matitis nodularis chronica helices).
4 Pinna haematoma (→ cauliflower ear).
5 Smooth, often multiple/bilateral swellings of the bony ear canals (exostosis) → build up of wax/debris → conductive deafness.
6 Wax (cerumen).
7 Foreign bodies in the ear.

Otitis externa (swimmer's ears):
1 Trauma.
2 Infection (pseudomonas; fungal).
3 Eczema.
4 Psoriasis.

Bullous myringitis:
1 Viral infection (influenza).
2 Bacterial infection (*Mycoplasma pneumoniae*).

Painful ear:
1 Otitis externa.
2 Furunculosis (boil in the meatus).
3 Malignant necrotising otitis externa.
4 Bullous myringitis.
5 Barotrauma (aerotitis).
6 Temporomandibular joint dysfunction.
7 Referred pain (from neck – C3, C4 and C5); throat infection; tooth problem).

Discharging ear:
1 Middle ear infection (ASOM with or without effusion; CSOM).
2 Cholesteatoma (locally destructive stratified epithelium).
3 External ear problem (chronic otitis externa; auditory canal trauma → bloody discharge).
4 CSF otorrhoea.

Otitis externa:
1 Hot climate (excessive sweating, bathing and swimming predispose to otitis externa).
2 Trauma.
3 Iatrogenic (ear syringing).
4 Skin disease (eczema or psoriasis of the external auditory canal).
5 Narrow or tortuous external auditory canal.

Acute otitis media:
1 Common cold.
2 Influenza.
3 Acute tonsillitis.
4 Coryza (of whooping cough, measles, scarlet fever).
5 Sinusitis.

Chronic otitis media:
1 Inadequatly treated/untreated acute otitis media.
2 Immunodeficient patient (any debilitating illness like CRF; steroid/cyto-toxic drug therapy; AIDS, etc).
3 Virulent infection.
4 Upper airway sepsis.

Otitis media with effusion (OME):
1 Inadequatly treated/untreated acute otitis media.
2 Nasopharyngeal obstruction (d/t large adenoids, nasopharyngeal tumour, etc).
3 Allergic rhinitis.
4 Barotrauma.
5 Idiopathic.

Epistaxis:
1 Spontaneous (from Little's area).
2 Hypertension.
3 Trauma/postoperative.
4 Coagulation defect (leukaemia; thrombocytopenia; anticoagulant therapy).
5 Hereditary haemorrhagic telangiectasia.

Deviated nasal septum (DNS):
1 Trauma (recent/old).

Nasal septal perforation:
1 Trauma (like nose-picking; postoperative especially following septal surgery [SMR; septoplasty]).

2 Systemic diseases (e.g. Wegener's granulomatosis; lupus; syphilis).
3 Basal cell carcinoma (rodent ulcer).
4 Cocaine addiction.
5 Inhalation of fumes of chrome salts.

Acute sinusitis:
1 Complication of other infection (e.g. common cold; influenza; measles; whooping cough) – the commonest cause.
2 Dental problem (dental extraction; apical abscess).
3 Swimming.
4 Fracture.

Chronic sinusitis:
1 Unresolved acute sinusitis (d/t anatomical anomaly, polyp, allergy or immunodeficiency).

Nasal polyposis:
1 Adult asthmatic who is aspirin sensitive.
2 Repeated URTI (d/t cystic fibrosis, Kartagener's syndrome, etc).

Acute tonsillitis:
1 Infectious mononucleosis.
2 Diphtheria.
3 Scarlet fever.
4 HIV.
5 Agranulocytosis.

Chronic laryngitis:
1 Excessive vocal use (as seen in teachers, actors, singers, etc).
2 Smoking.
3 Drinking spirits.
4 Chronic sinusitis.

Left recurrent laryngeal nerve palsy in the chest:
1 Iatrogenic (cardiac/oesophageal surgery).
2 Malignancy (ca. bronchus; ca. oesophagus; malignant enlargement of the mediastinal lymph nodes).
3 Aortic aneurysm.

Right/left recurrent laryngeal nerve palsy in the neck:
1 Iatrogenic (thyroid surgery; mediastinoscopy; cervical spine surgery).
2 Malignancy (ca. thyroid; ca. cervical oesophagus; ca. hypopharynx).
3 Penetrating neck injury.

Bilateral recurrent laryngeal nerve palsy:
1 Iatrogenic (thyroid surgery).
2 Malignancy (ca. thyroid).
3 Pseudobulbar palsy.

17 Obstetrics and gynaecology

Obstetrics:
Recurrent miscarriage:
1 Idiopathic in most cases.
2 Uterine abnormality (e.g. submucous myomata; uterine septa; endometrial infection).
3 Cervical incompetence.
4 Polycystic ovarian disease.
5 Autoimmune disease (e.g. antiphospholipid syndrome; SLE).

Pre-term delivery:
1 Pre-term labour (placental abruption; sepsis; idiopathic).
2 Elective delivery (pre-eclampsia; severe haemorrhage d/t any cause; foetal compromise).
3 Cervical incompetence.

Cervical incompetence:
1 Idiopathic.
2 Damaged cervix d/t previous surgery.
3 Secondary to congenital uterine anomaly.

Antepartum haemorrhage:
1 Placental problem (placenta previa; placental abruption; placental edge bleeding).
2 Cervical problem (cervicitis; cervical erosion; cervical polyp; cervical carcinoma).
3 Accidental haemorrhage.

Intrauterine growth retardation (IUGR):
1 Placental dysfunction (commonest cause).
2 Maternal disease (hypertension/pre-eclampsia (common); severe anaemia; poor intake; SLE).
3 Foetal problem (twins; transplacental infection; chromosomal/congenital anomaly).

Postpartum haemorrhage:
1 Atonic uterus (commonest cause).
2 Placental remnants.
3 Vulval/vaginal/cervical laceration.

4 Uterine dehiscence (d/t previous caesarean/myomectomy; forceps delivery).
5 Blood coagulation defect.

Secondary postpartum haemorrhage:
(24 hr to 6 weeks after delivery)
1 Retained placental remnants.

Hypertension in pregnancy:
1 Pregnancy-induced hypertension.
2 Pre-eclampsia.
3 Essential hypertension.

Coagulopathy in pregnancy:
1 Placental abruption.
2 Haemorrhagic shock (d/t any reason).
3 Septic shock.
4 Amniotic fluid embolism.
5 Retained dead foetus.

Polyhydramnios:
1 Idiopathic (most of the cases).

Foetal causes:
1 High urine output (macrosomia twin-to-twin transfusion).
2 Impaired swallowing of amniotic fluid (d/t a neuromuscular cause).
3 Regurgitation of amniotic fluid (d/t GI obstruction – oesophageal/duodenal atresia).

Maternal causes:
1 Diabetes mellitus.

Malpresentation:
1 Foetal problem (premature; congenitally anomalous; dead; twins).
2 Maternal pelvic problem (small pelvic inlet; SOL in the pelvis).
3 Liquor volume problem (polyhydramnios).

Puerperal sepsis:
1 Genital tract infection (wound infection; endometritis; salpingitis).
2 Urinary tract infection.
3 Breast infection.
4 DVT.

Gynaecology
Delayed menarche:
1 Constitutional (idiopathic delay in the activation of HPO axis).
2 Vaginal atresia.
3 Androgen insensitivity syndrome (46,XY karyotype; phenotypically female d/t peripheral resistance to androgens).

Menorrhagia:
1 Dysfunctional uterine bleeding (DUB) – commonest cause (no organic pathology present).
2 Systemic causes (hypothyroidism; bleeding diathesis).
3 Local uterine causes (submucous fibroid; endometriosis; endometrial polyp/carcinoma).
4 Pelvic inflammatory disease (PID).
5 IUCD.

Secondary amenorrhoea (absence of menstruation for ≥3 months):
1 Physiological (pregnancy; menopause).
2 Low body weight; anorexia nervosa; weight loss; exercise; stress.
3 Endocrine problem (hypopituitarism; post-pill pituitary insensitivity; hyperprolactinaemia; hypo- or hyperthyroidism).
4 Ovarian problem (PCOS; primary ovarian failure).
5 Uterine problem (Asherman's syndrome, i.e. intrauterine adhesions).
6 Adrenal pathology (congenital adrenal hyperplasia; Cushing's syndrome; androgen-secreting adrenal tumour).
7 GI pathology (coeliac disease).

Intermenstrual/postcoital bleeding:
1 Cervical/uterine polyps/ca.
2 Combined OCPs or HRT.
3 Endometritis; endometrial polyp/carcinoma.

Postmenopausal bleeding:
1 Endometrial carcinoma.

Vulval swellings:
Infective:
1 Viral infections (herpes simplex type II; warts;[1] molluscum contagiosum).
2 Bacterial infections (vulval abscess; Bartholin's cyst/abscess – caused by blocked duct).
3 Fungal infection (thrush caused by *Candida albicans*).

---

1 Also called condylomata acuminata d/t human papilloma virus.

Non-infective:
1 Hernia.
2 Lipoma.
3 Tumour.

Vulval ulcers:
Infective causes.
1 Viral infections (herpes simplex type II; warts; molluscum contagiosum).
2 Bacterial infections (vulval abscess; Bartholin's cyst/abscess – caused by blocked duct).
3 Fungal infection (thrush caused by *Candida albicans*).

Pruritus vulvae:
1 Vaginal infection (candidiasis; trichomoniasis).
2 Emotional problems.
3 Skin disease (psoriasis; lichen planus; leucoderma; intertrigo; scabies; allergic dermatitis).

Lumps in the vagina:
1 Cystocoele; urethrocoele; rectocoele; enterocoele.
2 Uterine prolapse.
3 Vaginal ca.

Ulcers and lumps in the cervix:
1 Cervical ectropion.
2 Nabothian cysts.
3 Cervicitis.
4 Cervical polyps; cervical intraepithelial neoplasia (CIN); cervical ca.

Vaginal discharge:
1 Excessive normal secretion.
2 Vaginitis (bacterial vaginosis; trichomonas vaginitis; monilia vaginitis).
3 Cervicitis (gonococcal cervicitis; chlamydial cervicitis).
4 Foreign body.
5 Cervical ectropion (erosions).
6 Endometrial polyp; ca. cervix.

18 Paediatrics

Rash – scalp:
1 Seborrhoeic dermatitis.
2 Eczema.
3 Psoriasis.
4 Infection (fungal).

Rash – mucous membrane:
1 Measles.
2 Herpes.
3 Kawasaki's disease.
4 Stevens–Johnson's syndrome.

Rash – flexor surfaces (antecubital and popliteal fosse):
1 Eczema.

Rash – extensor surfaces:
1 Psoriasis.
2 Henoch–Schönlein's purpura.

Rash – web spaces:
1 Scabies.

Rash – shin:
1 Erythema nodosum.

Failure to thrive:
1 Inadequate food intake (insufficient breast milk; wrong technique; too diluted bottle milk; no food other than milk; can't take food d/t cleft palate, cerebral palsy, etc).
2 Vomiting.
3 Malabsorption (coeliac disease; cystic fibrosis; protein-losing enteropathy).
4 Abnormally increased energy requirements (any chronic illness like chronic renal or heart failure).
5 Psychosocial deprivation.

Limp in 1–2-yr-old:
1 Trauma.
2 Septic arthritis/osteomyelitis.

3 Congenital dislocation of the hip.
4 Cerebral palsy.

Limp in 3–10-yr-old:
1 Trauma.
2 Septic arthritis/osteomyelitis.
3 Irritable hip (transient synovitis).
4 Perthes' disease.
5 Malignant deposit in the bone (leukaemia).

Limp in >10-yr-old:
1 Trauma.
2 Septic arthritis/osteomyelitis.
3 Juvenile idiopathic arthritis (JIA).
4 Slipped upper femoral epiphysis.
5 Osgood–Schlatter's disease.

Generalised lymphadenopathy:
1 Infection (CMV; infectious mononucleosis; rubella; toxoplasmosis; HIV).
2 Malignancy (leukaemia; lymphoma).
3 Juvenile chronic arthritis (JCA).
4 Kawasaki's disease.

Cervical lymphadenopathy:
1 Infection in the area of drainage.
2 TB.
3 Malignancy (lymphoma; neuroblastoma).

Short stature:
1 Familial; Turner's syndrome; constitutional delay; emotional deprivation.
2 Endocrinopathy: GH deficiency; hypothyroidism; Cushing's syndrome; steroid therapy.
3 Rheumatological pathology: achondroplasia; vitamin D-resistant rickets.
4 GI pathology: coeliac disease.
5 Any chronic illness: chronic renal/heart failure; cystic fibrosis, etc.

Late unsupported walking (i.e. after 18 months):
1 Familial.
2 Congenital dislocation of the hip.
3 Duchenne's muscular dystrophy (only in boys).
4 Cerebral palsy.

Ambiguous genitalia:
1 Congenital adrenal hyperplasia (CAH).

Congenital heart disease:
1 Down's syndrome (atrioventricular septal defect).
2 Turner's syndrome (AS; coarctation of aorta).
3 Congenital rubella (PS; PDA).
4 Alcoholism (ASD; VSD).

Hydrocephalus:
Non-communicating hydrocephalus (intraventricular obstruction):
1 Aqueduct stenosis.
2 Ventriculitis/ventricular haemorrhage.

Communicating hydrocephalus (extraventricular obstruction):
1 Tuberculous meningitis.
2 Subarachnoid haemorrhage.
3 Arnold–Chiari's malformation.

Cerebral palsy:
Antenatal problem (commonest cause):
1 Cerebral dysgenesis.
2 Antenatal infection (CMV; rubella; toxoplasmosis).

Intrapartum problem:
1 Birth asphyxia.

Postnatal problem:
1 Head injury.
2 Meningitis/encephalitis.

Wheeze in a child:
1 Bronchial asthma.
2 Inhaled foreign body.

19 Procedures

Lumbar puncture – indications:
Diagnostic:
  1 Fever with disturbed conscious level.
  2 Signs of meningeal irritation with or without fever.
  3 Unexplained coma.
  4 Suspicion of multiple sclerosis, acoustic neuroma, CNS involvement in lymphoma or leukaemia, GB syndrome or transverse myelitis.
  5 Myelography.

Therapeutic:
  1 Spinal anaesthesia.
  2 Intrathecal methotrexate in acute lymphoblastic leukaemia.

Lumbar puncture – contraindications:
  1 Papilloedema.
  2 Hypotension.
  3 Bleeding/clotting disorder.
  4 Local sepsis (use another site).

Lumbar puncture – complications:
  1 Infection.
  2 Low-pressure headache (if large quantity of CSF is removed).
  3 Transtentorial or tonsillar herniation.

Bone marrow aspiration/biopsy – indications:
  1 Aplastic anaemia.
  2 Pancytopenia (d/t megaloblastic anaemia, hypersplenism, etc).
  3 Haematologic malignancy (leukaemia; staging of lymphoma; multiple myeloma).
  4 Myelofibrosis.
  5 PUO.

Echocardiography with Doppler flow study – information yielded:
Anatomical information:
  1 Heart size; size of each heart chamber; thickness of heart walls; wall aneurysms.
  2 Wall motion abnormalities (akinetic/dyskinetic segments). Stress echo (stress = exercise or dobutamine) detects transient wall motion

abnormalities d/t reversible cardiac ischaemia.
3 Valvular and septal defects (stenosis; prolapse; regurgitation).
4 Congenital anomalies.
5 Pericardial effusion and pericardial thickening.

Physiological information:
1 Volumes (systolic; diastolic; ejection fraction).

Exercise tolerance test (ETT) – indications:
1 To rule out IHD as the cause of chest pain.
2 Assessment of exercise tolerance following myocardial revascularisation (thrombolytic therapy; coronary angioplasty).

ETT – contraindications:
1 Recent MI (within a week).
2 Unstable angina.
3 Severe AS.
4 Decompensated heart failure.
5 Malignant HTN.

ETT – indicators of test termination:
1 Target heart rate achieved (i.e. 85% of maximum heart rate [= 220 – age]).
2 Red-flag symptoms develop (severe SOB/exhaustion; chest pain; fall in BP by >15 mmHg; syncope).
3 Red-flag ECG changes (ST depression of >2 mm; SVT; VT).

HIDA scan – information yielded:
1 Acute cholecystitis (gallbladder not seen; CBD seen).
2 Biliary leaks (post-traumatic; postoperative).
3 Patency of biliary–enteric shunt.
4 Choledochal cyst.
5 Paediatric patients (differentiation of biliary atresia and hepatitis in neonates; congenital anomalies of the biliary system).

Whole body bone scan – indications:
1 To rule out bony metastases.[1]

CT scan – information yielded:
1 Brain: differentiates b/w different intracranial lesions (haematoma; abscess; tumour; cyst; infarction).
2 Lungs: diagnoses emphysema, bronchiectasis and interstitial lung disease.

---

1 It is sensitive but not specific; increased uptake is also seen in fractures, osteoarthritis and Paget's disease.

3 Diagnoses mass lesions of mediastinum, lungs and abdomen.

MRI scan – information yielded:
1 Particularly good in cerebellar, spinal cord and joint pathologies.

Liver biopsy – indications:
1 Chronic liver disease (chronic hepatitis; cirrhosis).
2 Hepatic malignancy (hepatoma; HCC; lymphoma; metastases).
3 Unexplained hepatomegaly; unexplained deranged LFTs.
4 Assessment of drug therapy (antiviral therapy; steroids).
5 PUO.
6 Storage diseases (glycogen-storage disease; amyloidosis).

Liver biopsy – contraindications:
1 Prolonged PT (>3 sec over the control after 10 mg of I/M vitamin K).
2 ↓ platelet count (<80 × 10⁹/L).
3 Tense ascites.
4 Hydatid disease of the liver.

Liver biopsy – complications:
1 Haemorrhage (haemothorax; intrahepatic haematoma; haemobilia; haemoperitoneum).
2 Intrahepatic AV fistula.
3 Serous membrane inflammation (pleuritis; perihepatitis).
4 Infection (hepatic abscess; biliary peritonitis).
5 Puncture of surrounding organs (gallbladder; kidney; colon).

Coronary angiography – indications:
1 Chest pain/cardiomyopathy with uncertain cause; patients with suggestive history in whom IHD needs to be clearly excluded (e.g. pilots).
2 High-risk disease as indicated by non-invasive testing or clinical scenario (post-MI/postangioplasty angina; limiting stable angina not improving on adequate medical treatment).
3 Patients with aortic valve disease who present with chest pain (to rule out whether this pain is d/t coronary artery disease).
4 Old patients undergoing valvular surgery (to determine whether or not they require concomitant CABG surgery).
5 Heart failure patients in whom a surgically correctable lesion is found (e.g. MR; LV aneurysm).

Revascularisation in angina patients – indications:
1 Angina patients not improving on adequate medical treatment.
2 Exercise testing in angina patients suggestive of severe disease (early positive ETT; large exercise-induced defect on thallium scanning).

3 Post-MI angina (clinical or on non-invasive testing).
4 Coronary angiography showing left main coronary artery stenosis of >50% with or without symptoms, triple-vessel disease with LV dysfunction (as indicated by EF <50% or previous transmural infarction), or two-vessel disease with LV dysfunction or >90% proximal stenosis (especially of LAD).

Dialysis – indications:
ARF:
Clinical:
1 Renal encephalopathy; convulsions.
2 Pulmonary oedema; fluid overload unresponsive to diuresis.
3 Pericarditis.
4 GI bleeding.

Biochemical:
1 Urea >200 mg/dL.
2 Daily rise in urea >40 mg/dL.
3 Creatinine >10 mg/dL.
4 K^+ >7.5 mEq/L.
5 HCO_3^- <12 mmol/L.

CRF:
1 Long-term maintenance dialysis.
2 Preparing and waiting for renal transplant.

Water-soluble poisoning cases:
1 Ethanol; methanol.
2 Barbiturates.
3 Salicylates.

Haemodialysis – contraindications:
1 CVS (hypotension; recent MI; pericarditis).

Peritoneal dialysis – contraindications:
1 Late pregnancy.
2 Abdominal pathology (intra-abdominal abscess; peritonitis; ascites; umbilical hernia; recent abdominal surgery).

Upper GI endoscopy – indications:
Diagnostic:
1 To ascertain the cause of dysphagia.
2 To ascertain the cause of upper GI bleed (oesophageal varices, peptic ulcer, etc).

3 Reflux oesophagitis.
4 Acid peptic disease (APD).
5 Gastric outlet obstruction.
6 Upper GI malignancy.

Therapeutic:
1 Upper GI bleeding ($\rightarrow$ sclerotherapy/band ligation of oesophageal varices; treatment of bleeding peptic ulcer).
2 Stricture /achalasia ($\rightarrow$ oesophageal dilatation; placement of a prosthesis across a stricture).
3 Removal of foreign body.

Upper GI endoscopy – contraindications:
1 CVS (recent MI; uncontrolled heart failure).

Colonoscopy – indications:
Diagnostic:
1 Bleeding PR.
2 Suggestion of IBD.
3 Suggestion of colorectal ca.

Therapeutic:
1 Polypectomy.

Colonoscopy – contraindications:
1 CVS (recent MI; uncontrolled heart failure).

ERCP – indications:
Diagnostic:
1 CBD pathology (stones; stricture [benign; malignant]; choledochal cyst).
2 Pancreatic pathology (chronic pancreatitis; ca. pancreas).

Therapeutic:
1 Sphincterotomy followed by balloon or basket extraction of the CBD stones.
2 Stent placement across a benign or malignant stricture.[2]

ERCP – complications:
1 Haemorrhage.
2 Inflammation/infection (cholangitis; pancreatitis).

---

2   A special NG tube can also be used for this purpose.

Percutaneous transhepatic cholangiography (PTC) – indications:
Diagnostic:
  1 To determine the site and cause (stones; stricture) of biliary obstruction.

Therapeutic:
  1 To relieve biliary obstruction by percutaneous biliary endoprosthesis.
  2 Preop. external biliary drainage through a catheter to improve patient's condition.

Percutaneous transhepatic cholangiography (PTC) – complications:
  1 Haemorrhage.
  2 Infection (biliary peritonitis; septicaemia).

20 Miscellaneous

Pyrexia of unknown origin (PUO) – diagnostic features:
1 Illness of at least three weeks' duration.
2 Fever over 38.3°C/100.94°F on several occasions.
3 Diagnosis has not been made after three outpatient visits or three days of hospitalisation.

Pyrexia of unknown origin (PUO) – causes:
1 Infection (malaria; typhoid fever; TB – pulmonary/extrapulmonary; infective endocarditis; infectious mononucleosis; abscess – dental/intra-abdominal; amoebiasis; brucellosis; fungal infection).
2 Malignancy (leukaemia; lymphoma; renal/hepatic/colorectal ca.)
3 Connective tissue/autoimmune disorders (SLE; RA; rheumatic fever; temporal arteritis; Graves' disease; sarcoidosis; autoimmune hepatitis).
4 CNS pathology (encephalitis; CVA; brain tumour; hypothalamic dysfunction).
5 Pulmonary embolism.
6 Drugs.
7 Factitious fever.

PUO – investigations done in all cases:
1 Blood CP.
2 Urine RE.
2 CXR.
4 Peripheral blood film for MP.
5 Widal test; typhi dot test.
6 Tuberculin test.
7 Sputum examination.
8 Brucella antibodies.
9 ANA.
10 USG abdomen.

PUO – investigations done when some clinical clue is present:
1 Blood C/S.
2 Echocardiography.
3 Biopsy (liver; lymph node; bone marrow).

Complications of gastrectomy:
1 Early satiety.

2 Postprandial fullness.

3 Postprandial hypoglycaemia.

4 Dumping syndrome (40%).

5 Bacterial overgrowth → malabsorption (deficiencies of iron, folic acid, B_{12}, Ca^{2+}).

6 Gallstones.

7 Anastomotic ulcer.

8 Ca. of gastric remnant.

Mitochondrial chromosome disorders – maternally inherited:

1 MELAS.[1]

2 MERRF.[2]

3 Leber's optic atrophy.

Diseases with some mitochondrial chromosomal abnormality:

1 Diabetes mellitus.

2 Deafness.

3 Parkinson's disease.

4 Alzheimer's disease.

---

1   MELAS: mitochondrial encephalomyopathy + lactic acidosis + stroke-like episodes.

2   MERRF: myoclonic epilepsy with ragged red fibres.

Acronyms

AAA abdominal aortic aneurysm
ABO ABO (blood groups; refers to A, B and C antigens on red cell membranes)
ABPA allergic bronchopulmonary aspergillosis
ACEI Angiotensin-converting enzyme inhibitors
ACTH Adrenocorticotrophic hormone
ADH Antidiuretic hormone
AF Atrial fibrillation
AFB Acid-fast bacillus
AIDS Acquired immunodeficiency syndrome
AML Acute myeloid leukaemia
ANA Antinuclear antibody
ANCA Antineutrophil cytoplasmic antibody
ANF Atrial natriuretic peptide
AP Anteroposterior
ADPKD Autosomal dominant polycystic kidney disease
APD Acid peptic disease
APTT Activated partial thromboplastin time
AR Aortic regurgitation
ARC AIDS-related complex
ARDS Acute respiratory distress syndrome
ARF Acute renal failure
ARVC Arrhythmogenic right ventricular cardiomyopathy
AS Aortic stenosis
ASAP As soon as possible
ASD Atrial septal defect
ASO Antistreptolysin O (titre)

ASOM Acute suppurative otitis media
ASOT Antistreptolysin O titre
AST Aspartate transaminase
ATN Acute tubular necrosis
AV Atrioventricular
AVM Arteriovenous malformation
BMI Body mass index
BOO Bladder outlet obstruction
BP Blood pressure
BPH Benign prostatic hyperplasia
BPPV Benign paroxysmal positional vertigo
BSF Blood sugar fasting
BT Bleeding time
Ca Carcinoma
CABG Coronary artery bypass graft
CAH Congenital adrenal hyperplasia
CBD Common bile duct
CCF Congestive cardiac failure
CD Contact dermatitis
CFA Cryptogenic fibrosing alveolitis
CHF Congestive heart failure
CIN Cervical intraepithelial neoplasia
CJD Creutzfeld–Jakob's disease
CK Creatinine (phospho) kinase (also CPK)
CKD Chronic kidney disease
CLD Chronic liver disease
CLL Chronic lymphocytic leukaemia
CML Chronic myeloid leukaemia
CMV Cytomegalovirus
CNS Central nervous system
CO Carbon monoxide

COPD Chronic obstructive pulmonary disease
CP Cicatricial pemphigoid
CPK Creatinine phosphokinase
CPR Cardiopulmonary resuscitation
CRAD Chronic restrictive airway disease
CREST Calcinosis, Raynaud's, esophageal dysmotility, sclerodactyly, telangiectasia
CRF Chronic renal failure
CRP C-reactive protein
CSF Cerebrospinal fluid
CSOM Chronic suppurative otitis media
CT Computed tomography
CVA Cerebrovascular accident
CVP Central venous pressure
CVS Cardiovascular system
CXR Chest x-ray
DC Direct current
DH Dermatitis herpetiformis
DIC Disseminated intravascular coagulation
DIDMOAD Diabetes insipidus; diabetes mellitus; optic atrophy; deafness
DIP Distal interphalangeal (joint)
DKA Diabetic ketoacidosis
DLE Discoid lupus erythematosus
DM Diabetes mellitus
DNA Deoxyribonucleic acid
DNS Deviated nasal septum
DPG Diphosphoglycerate
DU Duodenal ulcer
DUB Dysfunctional uterine bleeding
DVT Deep venous thrombosis

EAG Excess anion gap
EBV Epstein-Barr virus
ECG Electrocardiography
ECT Electroconvulsive therapy
EEG Electroencephalogram
EF Ejection fraction
EM Erythema multiforme
EMF Endomyocardial fibrosis
EMV Eye (opening), verbal (response), motor (response)
ENT Ear, nose and throat
EPI Extended programme of immunization
EPS Electrophysiological studies
ERCP Endoscopic retrograde cholangio-pancreatography
ESR Erythrocyte sedimentation rate
ETT Exercise tolerance test
FSH Follicular stimulating hormone
FVC Forced vital capacity
GB Gallbladder
GBM Glomerular basement membrane (disease)
GCS Glasgow coma scale
GE Gastroenteritis
GH Growth hormone
GI Gastrointestinal
GIT Gastrointestinal tract
GN Glomerulonephritis
GORD Gastro-oesophageal reflux disease
GPE General physical examination
GRA Glucocorticoid-remediable aldosteronism
GTT Glucose tolerance test
GU Gastric ulcer
HA Haemophilia A
HAV Hepatitis A virus
HB Haemophilia B
HBV Hepatitis B virus
HCC Hepatocellular carcinoma
HCG Human chorionic gonadotrophin
HCV Hepatitis C virus
HDV Hepatitis D virus
HELLP *H*aemolysis, *e*levated *l*iver enzymes, *l*ow *p*latelets
HEV Hepatitis E virus

HHT Hereditary haemorrhagic telangiectasia
HIDA Hepatic immunodiacetic acid
HIV Human immunodeficiency virus
HLA Human leukocyte antigen
HOCM Hypertrophic obstructive cardiomyopathy
HONK Hyperosmolar nonketotic (diabetic coma)
HPF High power field
HPO Hypothalamic-pituitary-ovarian (axis)
HR Heart rate
HRT Hormone replacement therapy
HSMN Hereditary sensorimotor neuropathy
HSP Hereditary spastic paraplegia
HSV Herpes simplex virus
HTN Hypertension
HUS Haemolytic uraemic syndrome
IBD Inflammatory bowel disease
IBS Irritable bowel syndrome
ICP Intracranial pressure
ICS Intercostal space
ICU Intensive care unit
IFG Impaired fasting glucose
IGF Insulin-like growth factor
IGT Impaired glucose tolerance
IHD Ischaemic heart disease
INH Isoniazid
INR International normalised ratio (prothrombin ratio)
IP Interphalangeal (joint)
ITP Idiopathic thrombocytopenic purpura
ITU Intensive treatment unit
IU International unit
IUCD Intrauterine contraceptive device
IUGR Intrauterine growth retardation

IV Intravenous
IVC Inferior vena cava
JCA Juvenile chronic arthritis
JIA Juvenile idiopathic arthritis
JVP Jugular venous pressure
KCO Corrected carbon monoxide (transfer factor)
LAD Left axis deviation (on ECG)
LBBB Left bundle branch block
LCM Left costal margin
LDH Lactate dehydrogenase
LDL Low-density lipoprotein
LE Lupus erythematosus
LGL Lown–Ganong–Levine's (syndrome)
LH Luteinizing hormone
LIF Left iliac fossa
LLQ Left lower quadrant
LMN Lower motor neuron
LP Lumbar puncture
LQTS Long QT syndrome
LRT Lower respiratory tract
LRTI Lower respiratory tract infection
LUQ Left upper quadrant
LV Left ventricular
LVF Left ventricular failure
LVH Left ventricular hypertrophy
MAHA Microangiopathic haemolytic anaemia
MAT Multifocal atrial tachycardia
MCGN Mesangiocapillary glomerulonephritis
MCT Medullary carcinoma thyroid
MCTD Mixed connective disorder
MCV Mean cell volume
MELAS *M*itochondrial *e*ncephalomyopathy, *l*actic *a*cidosis, *s*troke-like episodes
MEN Multiple endocrine neoplasia
MERRF *M*yoclonic *e*pilepsy with *r*agged *r*ed *f*ibres
MI Myocardial infarction
MND Motor neuron disease

MNG Multinodular goitre
MP Malarial parasite
MPO Myeloperoxidase
MR Mitral regurgitation
MRI Magnetic resonance imaging
MRSA Methicillin-resistant *Staphylococcus aureus*
MS Mitral stenosis
MSH Melanocyte stimulating hormone
MVP Mitral valve prolapse
NADH Nicotinamide adenine dinucleotide hydrogenase
NICE National Institute for Health and Clinical Excellence
NLD Necrobiosis lipoidica diabeticorum
NO Nitric oxide
NSTEMI Non-ST-elevation myocardial infarction
NVD Nausea, vomiting and diarrhoea
NYHA New York Heart Association
OA Osteoarthritis
OCP Oral contraceptive pill
OME Otitis media with effusion
PAN Polyarteritis nodosa
PBC Primary biliary cirrhosis
PCM Paracetamol
PCOS Polycystic ovarian syndrome
PCP Pneumocystis carinii (jiroveci) pneumonia
PCT Porphyria cutanea tarda
PDA Patent ductus arteriosus
PE Pulmonary embolism
PEFR Peak expiratory flow rate
PEM Protein-energy malnutrition
PG Pemphigoid gestationis
PID Pelvic inflammatory disease
PIP Proximal interphalangeal joint(s)
PMF Progressive massive fibrosis
PND Paroxysmal nocturnal dyspnoea
PP Postprandial
PR Pulmonary regurgitation

Per-rectum
Pulse rate
PR (interval on ECG)
PRP Pityriasis rubra pilaris
PS Pulmonary stenosis
PSC Primary sclerosing cholangitis
PT Prothrombin time
PTC Percutaneous transhepatic cholangiography
PTH Parathyroid hormone (parathormone)
PUO Pyrexia of unknown origin
PV Pemphigus vulgaris
PVD Peripheral vascular disease
QR QR (complex on ECG)
QRS QRS (complex on ECG)
QS QS (complex on ECG)
QT QT (interval on ECG)
RA Right atrium
RBBB Right bundle branch block
RBC Red blood cell
RBS Random blood sugar
RE Routine examination
RIF Right iliac fossa
RLQ Right lower quadrant
RNA Ribonucleic acid
RNP Ribonucleoprotein
RS RS (complex on ECG)
RSV Respiratory syncytial virus
RTA Renal tubular acidosis
RUQ Right upper quadrant
RV Right ventricle
RVF Right ventricular failure
RVH Right ventricular hypertrophy
SA Sinoatrial (node)
SAH Subarachnoid haemorrhage
SBP Spontaneous bacterial peritonitis
SIADH Syndrome of inappropriate ADH (secretion)
SJS Stevens-Johnson syndrome
SLE Systemic lupus erythematosus
SMR Submucous resection
SOB Shortness of breath
SOL Space-occupying lesion

SSSS Staphylococcal scalded skin syndrome
ST ST (segment on ECG)
STEMI ST-elevation myocardial infarction
SVC Superior vena cava
SVT Supraventricular tachycardia
TB Tuberculosis
TBG Thyroid-binding globulin
TCA Tricyclic antidepressants
TEN Toxic epidermal necrolysis
TFT Thyroid function test
TIA Transient ischaemic attack
TIBC Total iron-binding capacity
TLC Total leukocyte count
TLCO Total lung carbon monoxide (transfer factor)
TPN Total parenteral nutrition
TPO Thyroid peroxidase
TR Tricuspid regurgitation
TS Tricuspid stenosis
TSH Thyroid stimulating hormone
TSS Toxic shock syndrome
TT Thrombin time
TTP Thrombotic thrombo-cytopenic purpura
UMN Upper motor neuron
URT Upper respiratory tract
URTI Upper respiratory tract infection
USG Ultrasound
UT Urinary tract
UTI Urinary tract infection
UV Ultraviolet
VA Visual acuity
VDRL Venereal disease research laboratory (syphilis serology)
VF Ventricular fibrillation
VR Vocal resonance
VSD Ventricular septal defect
VT Ventricular tachycardia
VZV Varicella-Zoster virus
WHO World Health Organization
WPW Wolff–Parkinson–White's (syndrome)
XY XY (chromosomes)

Index